Praise for *The Emotionally Healthy Child*

"*The Emotionally Healthy Child* is a wonderful addition to the growing library of resources for parents and educators about the critical importance of understanding what emotional health looks like in the young. Maureen Healy provides us with clear and simple strategies to help children 'use the "dirt" of their daily experiences and steer toward the lotus of their lives.' In doing so, she provides a manual for 'progress without perfection.' A real gift."
— *Claire Kelly,* director of Mindfulness in Schools Project (MiSP)

"Maureen Healy provides simple yet life-changing tools to raise more mindful children."
— *Dr. Saamdu Chetri,* former director of
Gross National Happiness for Bhutan

"At last, a brilliant road map of what emotional health in children *is,* along with amazingly accessible tools of emotional coaching to help them get there. Generously filled with real-life examples and learning scenarios any parent, teacher, or coach can relate to, plus exercises to teach the necessary skills, this book is a real gift."
— *Linda Graham, MFT,* author of *Bouncing Back:
Rewiring Your Brain for Maximum Resilience and Well-Being*

"*The Emotionally Healthy Child* provides practical advice that is both accessible and potentially transformative — for the child, the parent, and their relationship. Read it, read it again, and then, more importantly, apply it."
— *Tal Ben-Shahar, PhD,* author of
Happier: Learn the Secrets to Daily Joy and Lasting Fulfillment

"*The Emotionally Healthy Child* can help any adult who wants to raise healthier and ultimately happier children in today's world."
— *Michele Borba, EdD,* author of *UnSelfie:
Why Empathetic Kids Succeed in Our All-About-Me World*

THE
EMOTIONALLY
HEALTHY
CHILD

Also by Maureen Healy

Growing Happy Kids

The Energetic Keys to Indigo Kids

THE
EMOTIONALLY
HEALTHY
CHILD

Helping Children
Calm, Center, and Make
Smarter Choices

MAUREEN HEALY

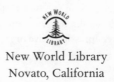

New World Library
Novato, California

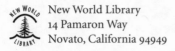

New World Library
14 Pamaron Way
Novato, California 94949

Text design by Tona Pearce Myers

Library of Congress Cataloging-in-Publication Data
Names: Healy, Maureen, [date]– author.
Title: The emotionally healthy child : helping children calm, center, and make smarter choices / Maureen Healy.
Description: Novato, Calif. : New World Library, [2018] | Includes bibliographical references and index.
Identifiers: LCCN 2018020624 (print) | LCCN 2018023482 (ebook) | ISBN 9781608685639 (ebook) | ISBN 9781608685622 (alk. paper)
Subjects: LCSH: Emotions in children. | Child rearing.
Classification: LCC BF723.E6 (ebook) | LCC BF723.E6 H43 2018 (print) | DDC 155.4/124—dc23
LC record available at https://lccn.loc.gov/2018020624

First printing, October 2018
ISBN 978-1-60868-562-2
Ebook ISBN 978-1-60868-563-9
Printed in Canada on 100% postconsumer-waste recycled paper

New World Library is proud to be a Gold Certified Environmentally Responsible Publisher. Publisher certification awarded by Green Press Initiative. www.greenpressinitiative.org

10   9   8   7   6   5   4   3   2   1

Keep me away from the wisdom which does not cry, the philosophy which does not laugh, and the greatness which does not bow before children.

KHALIL GIBRAN

CONTENTS

INTRODUCTION

Our parents bring us into the world, but in the end, we are responsible for what we become.

KHALIL GIBRAN

I was a wild child. The type of child whose family members would babysit and leave wondering whether they really wanted children. Of course I had my charms, but my energy was boundless. I could run circles in the backyard, climb up the weeping willow, take the dog for a walk, and then come home to make my own beaded barrettes. I was constantly in motion. Later on, we discovered that I had many allergies, and once those were addressed, my body came back into balance and I calmed a great deal.

But my emotions were still big and intense. I was also a highly sensitive child who cried when someone teased me or when I fell off the swing and scraped my knee. I felt things deeply and didn't know what to do with my big emotions. Luckily I found constructive outlets for my energy, such as gymnastics, piano, and tap-dancing, into which I could pour my emotional ups and downs. But these creative classes felt like temporary relief. Now I know that what I needed was to learn about emotions and what my role was in creating happier ones.

The ideas and tools in this book are what my younger emotional self was seeking — an understanding of how emotions work and how I could create better-feeling ones. Today's children are seeking the same things, and this book was born to address that need. My child clients have big feelings and face the same quandaries I had so many years ago, but fortunately they have me to guide them and provide them with activities that work, even in today's digital world.

People say to me, "I'm glad I grew up before the Instagram world put my awkward photos online," and I agree, but in some ways life is easier now. Information about how to feel happier and become emotionally healthy is now more accessible, which is a huge improvement over when I grew up playing Atari in my basement and not having a clue about what to do with my big emotions when I lost at Pac-Man.

One Big Idea

Emotional health is based on the ability to make better choices, even when feeling anger or another big emotion. Children and adults alike can learn how to identify their emotions, and then use the tools of emotional health to:

- stop
- calm
- make a smarter choice

These three simple steps have the power to change everything. One of the challenges of emotions is that the tricky or challenging ones usually have speed, and to stop requires skill and practice. Just saying, "Stop that" isn't enough to slow a fast-moving car; one needs to know how to apply the emotional brakes, come to a stop, and then move in another direction. This is what this book teaches.

Using the tools in this book, children and adults alike can learn to pay attention and catch themselves before they make not-so-smart choices. Adults often know a not-so-smart choice when we make one, whether it's screaming at someone or speeding twenty miles above the speed limit, so learning how to calm and center, and then make a smart choice, is not just good for your health — it's good for everyone around you. I define a *smart choice* as one that is good for you and good for others.

In this book, we explore this simple yet life-changing idea that we can become more mindful and then, with emotional knowledge as well as some new tools, make better choices. The types of choices that bring healthier and happier experiences into our lives and that allow us to model this uplifted life to our children and teach them how to do the same.

How This Book Helps

We may know what emotional health looks like, but often we don't know how to get there. This book will help you with the *how*. The how is where we struggle. As adults we can often identify what we want, whether it's a bigger home or happier children, but we need some guidance on how to go about achieving these things.

In *The Emotionally Healthy Child*, I show you how to teach children to master their emotions and move forward on their unique paths toward wholeness. Specifically, I share the:

- *Mindset*. The ideas that help children master their emotions and move them toward creating an emotionally healthy mindset.
- *Habits*. The practices that children can do both with and without you to help them calm, center, and make smarter choices.

Although it may sound like I'm giving you more to do, I'm actually not. I am asking you to spend the same amount of time with your children but to make this time more effective at certain moments when you can guide your children to learn new ideas and tools to bring them back into emotional balance.

In this book I explain that emotional health is the skill of balance. Coming back into emotional balance is something we learn and relearn throughout our lives, but today's children who can gain ideas, tools, and insight on how to do this can have a smoother ride on their journey by avoiding some unnecessary bumps. And even if they do hit a snag, they will have the tools and awareness to emerge stronger, healthier, and ultimately, whole.

Stronger Together

If you want to go fast, go alone. If you want to go far, go together.

AFRICAN PROVERB

What I know for sure is when we join together to learn and then teach our children how to become their emotionally healthiest selves, we're stronger. We create a community of like-minded adults committed not only to helping our children change their undies but also to steering their minds toward making smart emotional choices.

Because the more children can calm, center, and make a smart choice when feeling a big emotion, the more harmonious this planet will be. Instead of the norm being to react to their feelings in unskillful ways, such as pushing other children on the playground, the new norm becomes children taking mindful moments and making more conscious choices.

Part One

EMOTIONAL LEARNING

Chapter One

TODAY'S CHILDREN

We all want to raise emotionally healthy children. There's not one parent alive who wants to raise an insecure, sad, and isolated child. But the question is always: How can we do it?

Jenna threw a chair across the room in her third-grade class; Oscar was suspended for dropping the f-bomb in first grade; Leo refuses to do his daily homework; and every night Maggie has a screaming match with her mom about bathing. Being a parent or teacher isn't an easy role, but today's children are more intense, reactive, and emotional than ever before.

So the question becomes: How do we transform these challenges into something better? It's the opportunity of a lifetime.

Last summer I had the opportunity to visit one of the most beautiful gardens on the planet: Lotusland in Santa Barbara, California. Arriving on a sunny day, I was delighted to find the lotuses in bloom, and I was awestruck by these gorgeous flowers. Every lotus seed had to go through the dirt to become what I was able to behold. The same is true for children (and for you and me).

Helping children use the "dirt" of their daily experiences and steer toward the lotus of their lives is the focus of this book. I don't talk about pie-in-the-sky emotional health but real well-being that has grown from challenging moments. Said differently, a large part of becoming emotionally healthy is learning how to skillfully be with uncomfortable emotions and constructively express them. Maggie, for example, isn't screaming nightly anymore and has learned how to talk through problems more.

But that's not the whole enchilada. Children can also learn how to choose their thoughts and do the things that create emotional health. (Of course, those things might make you feel good, too.) In this book I share the path to children's positive emotional health and give you the tools to make healthier and happier a possibility, not just a pipe dream. Because ultimately when you're raising an emotionally healthy child, the world becomes better, too.

Emotional Health

It is very important to understand that emotional intelligence is not the opposite of intelligence, it is not the triumph of heart over head — it is the unique intersection of both.

DAVID CARUSO

Earlier today Carla, a mother of three, contacted me from Spain. She was seeking help with her ten-year-old son, Mateo, who has been having a lot of tears at school. "My husband and I are out of tools to help Mateo," explained Carla. Of course, this is a common feeling among parents, and probably why you picked up this book in the first place. What can you do? How do you teach your child self-control? What makes sense to a growing mind? What constitutes an emotionally healthy child?

Let's first define an emotionally healthy child, which will focus our minds and steer us toward our goals. The emotionally healthy child is learning to:

- name emotions (in self and others)
- express emotions constructively (not suppress them)
- use self-control
- respond versus react
- make smarter choices, even when challenged

Emotionally healthy children aren't perfect boys and girls; they're simply learning how to master their emotions and *gain emotional balance in their lives*. For example, Mateo has been crying when he gets frustrated at school, loses at the game Uno, and needs to transition from playing soccer to doing his homework. He hasn't yet learned how to regulate his emotional responses, but I know that with some understanding of how emotions work and some access to practical tools, he can make choices that feel better for him — as well as others.

Putting your child on the path of emotional progress is a large part of what positive parenting is all about. There is nothing wrong with Mateo crying if that's what he needs to do, but I want him to make a deliberate choice instead of simply having a knee-jerk reaction. Whether your child has a challenge with her anger or his sadness, the ability to identify emotions and begin to channel them into appropriate outlets is the mark of a child becoming emotionally aware, which is the first step toward positive emotional health.

Bravery with Emotions

I feel like my secret magic trick that separates me from a lot of my peers is the bravery to be vulnerable and truthful and honest.

KATY PERRY

Emotionally healthy children are learning to be brave. These boys and girls are becoming adept at standing up to their enemies and, maybe even harder, their friends. Or sharing their truth, as singer Katy Perry mentions in the quote above. But bravery underlies children's emotional health, since it takes an inwardly strong, courageous, and brave child to:

- overcome knee-jerk reactions
- face his or her intensity
- learn how to do things differently
- display self-control

Any person on the planet who musters the courage to face uncomfortable emotions such as jealousy, disappointment, rejection, loss, betrayal, or disgust is brave. But children's feelings tend to be bigger, faster, and more intense, which means they need to gather even more courage to help them handle these epic emotions.

Caroline, age ten, is facing her father's illness. He has been diagnosed with an inoperable brain tumor and appears to be worsening. Caroline is in the fifth grade, and her dad wants her to live a "normal life," so she picks herself up, goes to ballet class, gets lots of hugs from her friends, and connects with me weekly to help manage her emotions. Of course, she's feeling fear, anger, sadness, loss, and many more emotions, but underneath it I see a very brave girl facing her feelings instead of running from them. Scenarios like Caroline's are difficult, but she's learning how to muster her courage and face her feelings in a healthy way.

The Emotional Brain

When a child is upset, logic often won't work until we have responded to the right brain's emotional needs.
DANIEL SIEGEL AND TINA BRYSON

As I listen to six-year-old Ruby's mom, Rachel, I consider her description in terms of my understanding of brain architecture and development. Her update for the week went like this: "Ruby is impossible. She won't give me any time on the phone. Yesterday I was speaking to my mom in Israel for Yom Kippur, and Ruby began writing notes: You're ignoring me. This is more than a minute. You don't love me. Why do I have to go to temple?"

What Rachel didn't understand is that Ruby was operating fully out of her right brain (the emotional part) and not at all out of her left brain (the logical part). Her mom asked her to give her a minute, which was a reasonable (left-brain) ask, and when a minute passed, Ruby got angry (right brain) and began to write her notes, which her mom shared with me. They were adorably misspelled. But Rachel didn't see the humor in the situation and became increasingly angry.

Understanding how most children operate helps us connect with them better, keep that connection, and guide them toward better choices and more integrated decisions. Rachel was operating from her logical left brain ("One minute, please") and Ruby was all emotional right brain ("I need you, Mom"), so they were literally *speaking different emotional languages.* But if her mom recognized Ruby's emotional needs first, and then helped her see that this was a temporary delay (and not denial), with practice Ruby could learn to do things differently (using both her right and left brain).

Helping our emotional (right-brain) children bring their reason and logic (left brain) into the decision-making equation earlier is central to raising emotionally healthy children. Throughout this book, I share strategies for helping our sons and daughters do this, especially strategies for slowing down the fast right brain and bringing the slower, more deliberate left brain online sooner.

TAKE NOTE

RIGHT BRAIN, LEFT BRAIN

Children begin life operating from their right brain and respond emotionally when their needs need to be met (for example, they think "I'm hungry" and they cry). This is normal and healthy. But a natural part of healthy maturation is learning how to use both the left (thinking) and right (feeling) parts of the brain in unison so that children can make the best choices.

Right brain: The part of the brain involved in creativity, spontaneous play, understanding symbolism, timelessness, emotions, and nonverbal communication.

Left brain: The part of the brain involved in making logical choices, solving math equations, completing time-based activities, following directions, and learning language, especially syntax and grammar.

The left brain comes online at approximately age four, which is why I begin working with children ages four and up. Before a child has the capability to reason, it's challenging to teach him or her the skills of emotional learning.

The Emotionally Healthy Child

The root of all health is in the brain. The trunk of it is in emotion. The branches and leaves are the body. The flower of health blooms when all parts work together.

KURDISH SAYING

Paulo, age nine, fainted at school. He face-planted, and when he came to, his face was bloody, which was a sight for everyone in the cafeteria to see. Sam, one of his best friends, got very upset. He asked to call his mom, and the school office manager gave him permission to do so.

Speaking to his mom, Sam admitted he was scared. He'd never seen anything like this and was worried it could happen again. His mom, Chloe, reassured Sam that Paulo would be okay and that sometimes challenging things happen. Sam was satisfied with this, but of course the goal is to help Sam learn to self-soothe and handle these big emotions on his own. The good news is that Sam didn't act out destructively with his feelings. He is learning how to handle his uncomfortable feelings constructively, and with practice, he'll be able to steer his own emotional ship.

Like Sam, the emotionally healthy child is learning how to:

- constructively express his emotions
- ask for help (when needed)
- develop healthy habits
- form a skillful mindset
- connect with others in a meaningful way

What the emotionally healthy child *doesn't do* is ignore or repress his emotions, pretend he's okay when he's not, tease someone else, use addictive behavior to cover unwanted feelings (for example, playing excessive video games or eating loads of candy), and take his anger out on his siblings or friends. If your child does these things it doesn't mean that your child is emotionally unhealthy, just that these are not the behaviors of positive emotional health.

Said differently, we're helping our children (and ourselves) move from unconscious behaviors or reactions to conscious, deliberate choices. Ideally, these choices are based on the wisdom of how emotions work and what's in our best interest as well as in the best interest of others.

TAKE NOTE

EMOTIONAL HEALTH CONTINUUM

Emotional health isn't an all-or-nothing proposition. It exists along a continuum. On one end there is negative emotional health, marked by harboring negativity, having quick reactions, and making careless choices that injure oneself or others. On the other end of the spectrum lies positive emotional health, marked by healthy habits, an intelligent understanding of emotions, careful choices, self-awareness, and awareness of others.

Of course, most people (including children) fall somewhere in the middle, where they're wrestling with some challenging emotions (jealousy, anger, sadness) yet they keep making progress and better choices. They're moving in the direction of feeling healthier and happier.

Positive emotional health isn't about feeling good all the time, either. It's about being an authentic person who feels his or her feelings, learns how to constructively express them (not hold on to them), and form healthy relationships, despite whatever challenges appear in the outer world.

Creating Emotional Health

To reiterate, the path toward positive emotional health is one of increasing a child's awareness of self and others *while building skills*, gaining understanding (knowledge turned to wisdom), and making smart choices (good for them and others). The more a child learns how to calm, center, and then make smart choices, the better overall outcomes will be. Very few good decisions are made when one is angry or agitated.

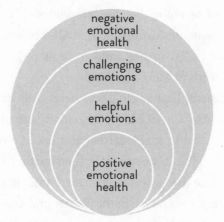

In the above image of emotional health, I don't address mental health disorders because someone can learn how to become emotionally healthier even while dealing with a disorder such as depression or anxiety. This is a dynamic model where we can all, hopefully, make sizable and positive gains in this lifetime.

Becoming more mindful is also part of positive emotional health, but that doesn't mean we need to be perfect. I've had plenty of moments when I was running on automatic and forgot to place postage on an envelope or couldn't find my keys (to later discover them in the freezer). Of course, they happen less and less, but life remains a wonderful adventure where some days just seem easier than others.

Connection to Happiness

Happiness is a form of courage.

GEORGE HOLBROOK JACKSON

Every emotionally healthy child is on the path toward happier experiences. She's learning to master her emotions and make choices that are good for her. Said simply, *emotional health is the first step toward becoming happier.* Happiness is complex, espe-cially if we're discussing lasting happiness. Of course, every parent and teacher wants his or her child to be happy, and this starts unequivocally with mastering emotions.

The emotionally healthy child isn't necessarily happy-go-lucky, but he is learning how to face his feelings in constructive ways. Jorge was the smallest kid in kindergarten, and because of this was an easy target for bullies. Unfortunately, the situation that his mom, Anna, feared came true when Jorge came home one day and said, "Momma, someone sat on me in the playground and punched me." Of the millions of questions that raced through his mom's mind, the one she asked was, "Did you tell anyone?" Jorge shook his head no.

Children like Jorge need to learn to speak up, especially when upset and scared. It takes a brave child to ask for help, which is what Anna is coaching her son to do. On my recommendation, she's get-ting him into jujitsu so he can feel physically as well as mentally and emotionally equipped to handle challenges like the bully at recess. While I'm not a fan of physical fighting, self-defense is necessary, and Jorge's confidence (inner and outer) will surely rise with some martial art skills under his belt (pun intended).

Becoming happier is the result of many things, but in this book we're beginning with mastering emotions and making smart choices (ones that are good for you and good for others).

Happier Comes from Challenges

Out of suffering have emerged the strongest souls; the most massive characters are seared with scars.

KHALIL GIBRAN

In his book with Desmond Tutu, *The Book of Joy,* His Holiness the fourteenth Dalai Lama talks about "passing through difficulties" and using them. He doesn't suggest being in a difficult spot and setting up camp there but instead focuses on passing through difficulties. Since children haven't yet gained a wider perspective, they tend to see whatever is happening as final, whether it's someone calling them names on the soccer field or something far worse.

Our role as parents and professionals is to help children begin to see how they can use any life experience, even the most challenging ones, as a force for good. Of course, I can only say this because I've learned to do this myself, even through experiences in which I thought for sure that there was no good to be found. Eventually a light shines on the dark spot, and life is made new again.

Last summer I had the pleasure of helping an eleven-year-old boy, Finn, recover from being bullied repeatedly. His parents, Margaret and Joe, brought him to me because he was slumped over and sad. Finn's demeanor was a result of being scared silly about returning to school as a seventh grader, with all the same bullies from the sixth grade.

Working with Finn, I shared how I had been bullied in grade school and called names I cannot even say aloud, all because of my full lips. He couldn't believe it. Once children realize they're not the only ones in a situation or that someone else has traversed the same path, they feel hopeful and can move up the emotional scale.

Finn and I did a lot of talking, and I gave him the chance to tell his story about being bullied one more time. Finn looked miserable, and the thing that struck me about his stories was that he assumed they were all true, especially when someone called him "weak" on the soccer field. But he wasn't weak, and I guided him how to see his situation differently (to reframe his story, a skill we'll discuss later in the book). For example, I mirrored back to Finn all the different and extraordinary things he's done that took strength — from rowing in regattas on Lake Casitas to teaching an elective, Lego Creativity, to his peers.

Changing your perspective isn't necessarily easy, especially when you have a history of being mentally or physically beat up. But with time and tools, I helped Finn focus on the positive things happening now and got his parents alerted and partnering with the principal. Eventually he came around to feeling more capable of handling whatever was going to come up in seventh grade.

Today Finn is a different child. By learning how to constructively express his emotions instead of suppressing them (holding his sadness in) and by developing some habits of emotional health, he's become a happier child. But this happiness isn't separate from his sadness and challenges; one helped the other grow.

The Challenges of Childhood

The gem cannot be polished without friction, nor man perfected without trials.

CHINESE PROVERB

Being small and new to the world has its challenges. Some common challenges occur in childhood, regardless of where you live, what you look like, and who your parents are. Some of those intrinsic obstacles are:

- *Lack of experience.* Children believe that everything that's happening to them is the worst thing ever. They simply don't have the experience and wider perspective to realize what a real problem is (someone committing suicide) versus a temporary challenge (getting poison ivy). Of course, it is good news when children are innocent, but their lack of experience limits their ability to perceive things accurately.

- *Lack of knowledge.* Boys and girls often don't have the training needed to handle challenging emotions. For example, Jenna didn't know how to handle her intense anger, and she threw a chair across her classroom. Thankfully no one was hurt, but her act did land her in the principal's office. The good news is that when Jenna learned how to do things differently, there were no more chairs flying across her third-grade classroom.

- *Lack of choice.* Copper, age ten, was one of my Skype clients. One of the most memorable things he said was, "I feel trapped at school." He begged his parents to change schools and even to homeschool him, but they refused. Children like Copper often feel that they don't have a choice on a subject, or that their voice isn't being heard, which is challenging for them.

- *Incorrect perceptions.* Children tend to put things together that aren't related and then form what are called illusory correlations. For example, when five-year-old Maggie's grandmother died, she asked me, "What did my grandmother do wrong?" And I replied, "Nothing. She lived a long time, and it was her time to go back to spirit." Since Maggie noticed everyone was upset, she assumed her grandmother did something wrong and hence died, but as we know, life doesn't work that way.

- *Lack of logic.* Before age eight children often have a lot of magical thinking, which is part of play and creative development. With magical thinking, a child's developing brain does not yet differentiate fantasy from reality (the logical and linear world). For example, I remember jumping off a picnic table when I was a young girl, thinking I would land like Wonder Woman; but I didn't, and my wrist blew up like a balloon.

Being a young child is overwhelming, emotional, and sometimes amazing but often frustrating, because of needing to adhere to parents' or teachers' rules. Yes, the adults probably know better, but when you're young, you don't realize this. Sometimes you just feel misunderstood because you want to play video games and not be pestered about doing your homework. Part of being a child means you don't have the whole picture, and the challenges mentioned are inherent to the experience of growing up.

The Way Forward

Don't limit a child to your own learning, for he was born in another time.

RABINDRANATH TAGORE

Children who learn about their emotions, connect with others in healthy ways, and begin to correct misperceptions (in age-appropriate ways) will be more successful. When they begin to master their emotions, from frustration to exhilaration, they move forward on the path of progress. Without any emotional self-control, a child stays stuck in a cycle of reactions, mistakes, and unconscious behavior.

Ella, age eleven, was very upset when she called me. Her grandmother had been rushed into the emergency room, and her "best friend" Madison had been spreading rumors about her. Of course, I listened to all the details, and then I helped Ella see the situation differently, and it immediately shifted how she felt. When you're in sixth grade, you cannot see the big picture; you think Madison's rumor is the worst thing ever, and you immediately assume your grandmother is dying, which may not be the case.

Children like Ella who are learning how to handle uncomfortable emotions benefit greatly from emotional coaching and education. They need your support until they can begin processing these big emotions on their own and sail through challenges with an emotionally healthy mindset. In the meantime, this book equips you with information on:

- how emotions work
- strategies to help your children
- the mindset of emotional health
- mindfulness strategies

I titled chapter 6 "The Toolbox" because it is a directory of emotions and the tools or strategies that help children with them. Emotions range from feeling sad and stressed to feel-good feelings such as hope and enthusiasm. The goal is to provide you with an easy-to-use toolbox at your fingertips, which you can turn to repeatedly when you (or your child) needs guidance on how to handle a big feeling.

Up Next

In chapter 2 I share the big picture of raising an emotionally healthy child and help you focus on the big wins as well as the little steps as you move in a healthier direction.

Chapter Two

THE BIG PICTURE

We learn most readily, most naturally, most effectively, when we start with the big picture — precisely when the basics don't come first.

ALFIE KOHN

One of my most memorable family trips as a child was going to the Metropolitan Museum of Art in New York City. I fell in love with the Egyptian wing, seeing mummies and hearing the stories of the hieroglyphs and scribes, as well as seeing the artwork, especially the Impressionist paintings. Clear as day, I still remember standing in front of a Seurat painting (*A Sunday Afternoon on the Island of La Grande Jatte*) and being mystified. Up close, I couldn't make out the image. But as I slowly moved back, the forms came into view. Twenty feet away, I could see the painting beautifully.

Children's emotions are like this Seurat painting: when we view them up close, it's sometimes challenging to see what's happening, but with distance and time, things become clear. With emotional health, we need to take a step back to see the big picture before we can understand the key skills needed in a given situation. For example, Billy was in second grade, and his parents were getting messages from the principal daily about how their son was misbehaving. Knowing that children don't misbehave for no reason, I met with Billy and discovered that he himself was being bullied. He was taunted on the playground when no one was looking, but somehow the teacher only seemed to show up when Billy pushed or hit someone in retaliation.

School officials deemed Billy a "bad apple," based on his teacher's reports, but that wasn't the truth of the situation. Stepping back, we can see that Billy was being teased relentlessly, which the school didn't appreciate. They saw Billy as a behavior problem, which in the context of being teased daily is somewhat understandable, albeit still not acceptable. I could see Billy's pain and his need to learn how to navigate his challenging emotions and to get into a better environment.

Understanding the big picture of emotional health helped me advocate for Billy, build his skills of emotional health, and ultimately guide his family to move him to a new school, which made a huge and positive difference (no more calls from the principal).

Emotional Balance

Happiness is a skill, emotional balance is a skill, compassion and altruism are skills, and like any skill they need to be developed. That's what education is about.

MATTHIEU RICARD

Coming back into balance is at the core of emotional health. There is no greater joy or challenge on this planet, in my opinion, than learning how to master your emotions. And the good news is that we don't need to figure it out by ourselves. The way has already been made, which helps us see the big picture and have more compassion for our children as we take the smaller steps.

What is the big picture? To answer that question, I want to break down how I conceptualize emotional health:

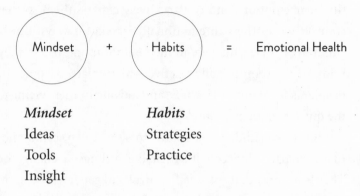

Mindset   +   Habits   =   Emotional Health

Mindset	*Habits*
Ideas	Strategies
Tools	Practice
Insight	

Emotionally healthy children are learning how to see the world, master their emotions, and use tools of emotional health as they come back into balance. They're building their emotional vocabularies, learning tools such as mindfulness, and developing the critical skill of self-awareness.

In future chapters we will delve more deeply into what children need to know (chapter 3, "Ideas"), what children need to do (chapter 4, "Tools"), and what speeds up the process of emotional health (chapter 5, "Insight"). I will also share some emotional tools (chapter 6, "The Toolbox") to help you put these new ideas into practice.

My aim is never to give you more to do but simply to make the time you spend with your children more effective, as you love them into the fullness of who they are.

The Essential Skills

It is our responsibility to learn to become emotionally intelligent. These are skills, they're not easy, nature didn't give them to us — we have to learn them.

PAUL EKMAN

Emotionally healthy children aren't simply born — they are made. They're nurtured and taught skills that help them identify their emotions and constructively express them so they can connect with others in emotionally intelligent ways. But before children begin learning about their emotions in earnest, they typically are very emotionally reactive, which creates a ripple effect of problems for parents, teachers, and anyone in their vicinity, even the quiet-seeking neighbors.

But once children learn how to slow down, calm, and then make smarter choices with their big feelings, a change occurs. They learn how to display self-control and gain awareness of their varied emotions. On this journey, four big-picture skills will help your children become emotionally healthier, and they are the ability to:

1. pay attention
2. respond (versus react)
3. press pause
4. make a smart choice

Although these steps may sound simple, they're not necessarily easy. They take practice and patience from adults as well as children, but they're possible for every healthy child.

Paying Attention

The simple act of paying attention can take you a long way.
KEANU REEVES

Some moments require your full attention, from carrying the Thanksgiving Day turkey to the table to doing tree pose in yoga. But in truth, bringing our focus and attention to almost everything we do, which without judgment and with our complete presence is called mindfulness (more on this in chapter 5), can help us make smarter choices. The same is true for our children, especially regarding their emotions.

Jimmy, age five, gets a little annoyed when his younger sister, Eugenie, takes his toys. Then his irritation increases when his older brother, Jack, bumps him by accident and knocks down his bamboo blocks. Jimmy hasn't been in the habit of paying attention to his body and how it feels, so before you know it he is screaming bloody murder and stomping around the living room. This likely could have been prevented, but the question is, How?

The first step is helping Jimmy learn to tune in to the signs his body was giving him when he felt just a little annoyance before the big anger set in. He needs to spot his emotions when they're small and then learn to constructively express them. Other ways to express his feelings (besides screaming) could have been:

- talking to parents
- going outside to play
- speaking up for himself: "Please don't knock my toys down."

Granted, five is a young age to begin mastering emotions, but it's not impossible. Children this young are building their emotional vocabulary and learning to identify not only particular emotions and what they mean but where they're feeling them in their bodies (more on this in chapter 4). Helping Jimmy begin to spot a challenging emotion like anger when it's in its baby form (annoyances, frustrations, and irritations) is the starting point of awareness of that emotion.

As you will see, paying attention to how we feel is a theme running throughout this book. Although many emotionally reactive children start without this skill, they certainly can learn it.

TAKEAWAY

THOUGHTS CREATE FEELINGS

One emotional aha I experienced was when I realized that our thoughts create our feelings. When we think a new thought, we experience a new feeling. In Jimmy's case, he was probably (either consciously or subconsciously) thinking, "This isn't fair. My brother isn't nice to me. I can't be pushed around like this." As these thoughts gathered momentum, he became angry, resulting in his screaming. But if he learned to think a new thought sooner, such as, "No one can push me around. I'm going elsewhere to play. I am going to have fun, no matter what," then his emotions would not escalate into yelling and he would feel much better.

Many children, including ones as young as Jimmy, and adults get stuck in their thinking, which produces certain feelings. Some of those feelings aren't helpful, such as anger, disgust, and jealousy. Helping boys and girls shift their thoughts and thus produce more helpful feelings can move them toward positive emotional health and ultimately toward happier moments. It all begins with paying attention to how their bodies are feeling and the thoughts they are thinking.

Responding vs. Reacting

We cannot always control everything that happens to us in this life, but we can control how we respond.

L. LIONEL KENDRICK

Children are often emotionally reactive, with big feelings and quick reactions that aren't always pleasing to the eyes or ears. But with some guidance, most children can learn how to pay attention, stop, and respond from a calmer place instead of simply reacting carelessly. Developing the ability to stop, calm, and make a smarter choice is at the core of this book, but it is also at the heart of responding constructively versus reacting negatively.

Remember the scenario with Billy? Billy was considered the problem child for standing up for himself on the playground and pushing another child. He certainly could have done things differently, such as walked way, used his words, or told a teacher, but he was "emotionally hijacked" in the moment, and his brain became flooded with angry emotions. With some new ideas, tools, and practice, Billy has been able to respond versus react even when he's feeling challenging emotions. (Of course, he's not perfect, but he's moving in the right direction.)

The same can be said of our preschooler, Jimmy, whose mom, Beatrice, has been helping him name the feelings in his body when they're still small. They've been using one of my tools from chapter 4 (Tool 1, Volcano, on page 74), which helps identify angry feelings in the body when they're small and manageable versus the size of Hagrid from Harry Potter and nearly impossible to control. If you can spot an emotion when it's little, there is a better chance you will be able to catch the emotion and release it constructively.

Smarter choices often come from responding and not reacting. As we've been learning, a large part of raising an emotionally healthy child includes guiding him or her to slow down and pay attention, pause, and then respond from an intelligent place.

TAKE NOTE

FASTER IS NOT ALWAYS BETTER

Although "The Tortoise and the Hare" is a fable, like most fables, it does convey some truth. The fastest person doesn't necessarily finish first, and this is true when it comes to emotions. Studying emotions, especially emotional health and happiness, over the past ten years has taught me that conscious choices are far better than most speedy reactions. This often means slowing down to get somewhere sooner. Children have a natural tendency to move quickly and often need help slowing down. I remember my mother saying that I had two speeds: on and off. I was either climbing a tree in the backyard or taking a nap; there was no middle ground. With time and training, I learned how to have this middle ground, which is a more sustainable place to be and can lead toward real joy.

Pressing Pause

The real secret of freedom may simply be extending this brief space between stimulus and response.

DOUG ABRAMS

If we don't learn how to slow down and stop in the middle of habitual patterns or behavior, nothing changes. It's especially challenging if your son or daughter has clocked many hours reacting in a certain way, but change is possible for most children. (The exception would be the child who is clinically depressed or biologically compromised, which needs to be addressed first.)

Children have an easier time learning how to "press pause" when they have someone guiding them and modeling that behavior to them. This can be you, or it can be a mentor, coach, or therapist. The magic of mirror neurons is one of neuroscience's recent discoveries. Basically, in nonscientific terms, this means that in the presence of someone who has learned how to press pause (or any other skill), it becomes infinitely easier for you and your children to develop that same ability.

When Hazel, age six, gets frustrated with her math homework, instead of pressing pause, she's gotten into the habit of letting out her anger in not-so-helpful ways, such as saying mean things ("You hate me, Mom! You want me to be miserable!"), crying, and hitting her brother (the A-plus student). Hazel simply doesn't yet have the emotional tools to handle her big emotions skillfully.

Her mom, Clara, gets so frustrated that she yells at Hazel, and then Hazel gets upset because she's sincerely struggling with her homework. Doing a math assignment in which you count forward by five and then backward by five may sound simple to an adult, but for Hazel it is super challenging.

To help Hazel navigate her big emotions, and signal to her mom that she needs to press pause, especially so things don't escalate, I gave her some scripts to use:

- "I need to pause."
- "Mom, I need a mindful moment."
- "I am feeling frustrated. Can we stop for a few minutes?"

Children like Hazel need to feel empowered to speak up for themselves when they're feeling overwhelmed, and they often need the precise language so they know what to say. The good news is that it hasn't taken long for Hazel to get a handle on speaking up for herself. She is helping her mom get the signal when she needs to press pause and handle her emotions before she can proceed with her homework.

Avoid this: Hazel's parents rewarded her for getting 100 percent on her math homework, and if she got any wrong she wasn't rewarded. This isn't the best approach. Children need to be rewarded for their efforts and not necessarily their outcomes. If you reward a child only for outcomes such as As on tests, they seek outer validation and do not develop a growth mindset, a precursor to life success. To paraphrase Sir Winston Churchill, the child who can bounce back from one failure to the next without losing enthusiasm is learning how to be successful. But the child who needs 100 percent correct on math homework to feel valued is not learning this. This is a parenting faux pas that too many of us fall into.

TAKE NOTE

MIRROR NEURONS

Scientists studying mirror neurons have found that when we see someone being calm, we activate similar neurons in our bodies. This is revolutionary because it means we can learn to press pause faster by being with someone who has already learned to do so. An article in *Scientific American* explains that mirror neurons "collapse the distinction between seeing and doing." So a child who wants to learn to stop herself before reacting can learn to do so by seeing someone else do this.

This dovetails with my background in Buddhism; I was taught that you can learn in two ways: (1) formally in a classroom, or (2) by being in the presence of another. Mirror neurons seem to explain the idea of "catching an idea" by simply being with another person who already possesses the skill, quality, or wisdom you're seeking.

Making Smart Choices

Sometimes it's the smallest decisions that can change your life forever.

KERI RUSSELL

Children are constantly making choices — from what socks to put on to what friend to invite over for a playdate — but the choices I'm referring to are the emotional ones. What does your son do when he's overwhelmed? Does he scream or cry? Or does he go into his bedroom and write in his journal? Those are very different choices. Of course, there's nothing wrong with boys or girls crying, but the idea is for children to make conscious choices that honor their momentary experience and serve them in the long term.

As we've seen, the emotionally healthy child is learning how to make choices that are good for him or her and good for others, which I call *smart choices*. Since life is simply a sum of our choices, the earlier we teach our children how to make smart choices, which integrate the whole brain (right and left hemispheres), the more positive their life trajectory becomes.

So what does that really mean? It means that as a parent you are responsible not only for making sure your child changes her clothes but also for her learning how to change her mind, see the positive, slow down, and express her emotions constructively. It's really an enormous task, which is why I'm a huge proponent of social and emotional learning (SEL) in the classroom; research shows that it is children's emotional intelligence that helps them succeed in life.

Kate, a mother of two girls, contacted me about her eight-year-old daughter's choices. Marisa knows the family rule that at 7:00 AM the TV in her room must go off, which leaves her thirty minutes before they need to leave for school. Yesterday Marisa's dad, Mike, turned off the TV at 7:05 AM, and Marisa turned it back on again. Mike wasn't having this, and said, "This is not happening. You must turn the TV off and get ready for school. I'm not going to be late today."

Marisa instantly went into tears and screaming. She yelled at her dad, "You hate me" and "I hate you." The tears and screaming persisted for fifteen minutes. Kate tried to help her calm down, but Marisa was already emotionally hijacked and hadn't yet learned to create enough space between stimulus (anger) and response (tears, screaming, mean words) to make a different choice.

At this point we couldn't change how Marisa had already responded, but she can learn how to make smarter choices with her big feelings in the future, which includes:

- paying attention (catching the feeling when it's small)
- pressing pause
- responding versus reacting

Children like Marisa can learn how to pay attention to their feelings and stop before they release them in destructive ways. Of course, many children, like Marisa, have challenges disconnecting from screens, which we will discuss shortly.

As adults we also need to take responsibility for our choices and for how we connect with or disconnect from our children. Mike, Marisa's dad, took an authoritarian approach with his daughter (think: *My way or the highway*), and it backfired on him in the form of a tantrum. I suspect if he had emotionally attuned and connected to Marisa and helped her feel seen, she may have moved through her emotions easier. But maybe not — sometimes things just go off the rails, and we need to begin again. Eventually there's a day when instead of a breakdown, your child has a breakthrough, and this is what we're aiming for.

Avoid this: Marisa's dad lost his cool and became very angry. When we lose it and raise our voices, we give our children permission to do the same. So the more we learn how to stay sane, even in the stressful moments of getting the children out the door in the morning, the better we model positive emotional health. Of course, this doesn't mean we need to be perfect but simply honest, respectful, and authentic. And if we mess up (as we're bound to do), a sincere apology helps repair the parent-child relationship.

The Emotional Landscape

The voyage of discovery lies not in finding new landscapes,
but in having new eyes.

MARCEL PROUST

Our children feel things deeply, including surprise, delight, disgust, anger, frustration, revenge, jealousy, and enthusiasm. They
often don't even have the words to communicate their feelings,
which is why they sometimes act them out inappropriately, but
once they learn what emotions are and how they work, and apply
a method to release them constructively, they can experience
emotional ahas, which lead them in a positive direction.

We will delve into these topics in later chapters, but for now
I want to share how I conceptualize emotions, especially as I see
emotional health. There are two types of emotions:

1. helpful
2. challenging

When I work with children, we focus on cultivating the helpful emotions and an emotionally healthy mindset so that children
can see the world accurately and respond with intelligence. They
learn to use their right and left brain in unison as much as possible at their stage of emotional development. We also work on
identifying challenging emotions — let's not say negative or bad,
but those emotions that throw them off-balance, which they need
to release constructively.

Often we begin by helping our children with their challenging emotions, because those are the ones that literally scream the
loudest. Boys and girls yell, cry, and stomp their feet in anger,
sadness, and frustration. But it's the helpful emotions such as
patience, calmness, and enthusiasm that need to be equally culti-
vated to balance the scales and enlarge a child's capacity to handle
the challenging emotions.

Ultimately, your child doesn't need to be all smiles but must be able to face any emotion that arises and learn how to skillfully express it. This is the emotionally healthy child. He is learning to embrace his whole bucket of emotions and then empty it when he needs to. He also learns how to fill his bucket with positive relationships, interests, and activities, which give his life meaning and purpose.

The Secret to Success: Discomfort

If you're never able to tolerate a little bit of pain and discomfort, you'll never get better.

ANGELA DUCKWORTH

One of the biggest challenges to children becoming emotionally healthy is the fact that they often cannot tolerate discomfort. They feel an uncomfortable emotion like anger and immediately want it to be gone, so they scream, punch, or throw a tantrum to release it. This provides relief but isn't constructive. One of our roles in raising emotionally healthy children and helping them transform lemons into lemonade includes helping them:

- embrace discomfort
- increase their "discomfort tolerance" level
- realize that uncomfortable emotions come and go

Children can learn to raise their discomfort tolerance by feel uncomfortable in a safe environment. Fatima, age seven, wants to win at every board game she plays. She's a perfectionist by anyone's standards, which is why I introduced a game that was a little tough for her and which I thought she'd likely lose (a very uncomfortable emotion). And yes, she did lose at the board game, *Clue*, which incited some distressing emotions, but I helped her work through them and realize that she was bigger than any challenging emotion.

When I was younger I recall my parents introducing me to novel experiences to widen my comfort zone, such as going to the Macy's Thanksgiving Day Parade in New York City, with millions of people, and visiting cousins in Ireland who didn't yet have indoor plumbing, so the bathroom was outside (what?). I learned early on that sometimes the really good things are at the other end of discomfort, and you need to go through the discomfort, not around it, to have unforgettable and happier experiences.

I'm not necessarily suggesting that you take your children to farms without plumbing, but I am suggesting that you help expand your children's ability to tolerate discomfort in safe and positive ways. This will also help them realize they are bigger than any of their big feelings. Children have the capacity to endure a little discomfort, express it constructively, and move beyond it to something more positive.

TAKE NOTE

CHILDREN'S BRAINS ARE STILL "COOKING"

Your child's brain isn't fully formed until his midtwenties, and the last thing to come online is judgment (in their prefrontal cortex). This is one of the best reasons to muster more compassion for your child, since he's not "fully cooked" yet. Children are learning not only how to bring logic (left brain) online sooner but also how to move from quick reactions (lower brain) to more deliberate responses (upper brain). Knowing that some of your child's challenges in becoming less reactive are biologically rooted, can help you find the patience to help him yet again. This includes helping him form new neuronal pathways, where he tolerates more discomfort and moves through it with inner confidence.

Wholeness, Not Happiness

Life is about more than happiness....It's okay to feel all the things we feel.

SCOTT STABILE

One of my passions in life is helping children become happier, whether they've lost a soccer game or something far more serious. The path to positive emotional health and happier experiences isn't around these challenges but through them. Whether the challenge is a bully on the bus or a bruised knee, every child has moments of sadness, anxiety, disappointment, and rejection when they just don't know what to do.

Our job is to be their cheerleaders, to help them rise up and move forward with skill on the path toward becoming emotionally healthy and happier. But make no mistake — my goal isn't simply to help you raise your children's happiness but something even more valuable: their wholeness, the ability to embrace whatever emotion is occurring, whether it's easy like joy or more challenging like grief. The whole child is learning to be honest, authentic, and genuine about her emotions.

Wholeness is important because it's based on the idea that all our emotions, helpful and challenging, are good and that it's what we do with them that matters. If your daughter is angry, she doesn't pretend everything is okay. She might say instead, "I feel rotten," and that is perfectly healthy. Being honest about our emotions, and learning how to express them constructively, is the mark of real emotional health, not simply putting on a happy face.

His Holiness the Dalai Lama is the happiest person I've had the honor to orbit near, as well as what I would consider a whole human being. He said, "I am sometimes sad when I hear the personal stories of Tibetan refugees who have been tortured or beaten. Some irritation, some anger comes. But it never lasts long. I always try to think at a deeper level, to find ways to console." His Holiness doesn't deny his anger or sadness but looks to use those feelings constructively. This is the highest octave of wholeness.

We want to raise healthier, happier, and yes, whole children. Boys and girls who can face emotions, become tolerant of uncomfortable feelings (anger, nervousness), and recognize that they're capable of handling whatever shows up. One of my clients, Simone, at age ten is learning how to face her challenging emotions. She's the main character in her upcoming school play, *The Sound of Music*, and has the jitters. Simone is learning relaxation techniques but also that being nervous is normal, especially if you've never done something before.

Being whole is valuable because it allows you to honor each moment, face whatever arises, and seek to be an authentic person who experiences all of life's different emotions without prejudice. Helping children learn not to run from their challenging feelings but to handle them with skill is a message that we'll return to throughout this book because it's necessary for every emotionally healthy child.

Bump in the Road: Screens

What I tell my kids is, "I'm preparing you for college and for life. So, having independence, knowing how to set your own boundaries, figuring out how to make that balance. We still have screen-time rules."

MICHELLE OBAMA

Last year I was asked to provide commentary after a group of parents watched the documentary *Screenagers* together. Sitting in the audience, I could hear audible gasps when doctors discussed how a scan of a child's video game–obsessed brain was similar to that of an adult drug addict. Both were seeking those immediate feel-good chemicals, dopamine and serotonin, which they felt when they got immediate satisfaction from the video game or the drug.

Certain personalities are more prone to addictive behavior, which is rooted in their genetic heritage and biological composition. Said differently, some children aren't even interested in playing video games, while another child cannot turn the game off without a screaming match. For the latter scenario, what is the solution? That's the million-dollar question, without one definitive answer, but research has shown that these approaches help:

- Create a media agreement (noting how much screen time is agreed on daily).
- Set rules.
- Model healthy disengagement (from devices).
- Praise progress.

Ultimately, you need to recognize and work with the child you have. My office has a waiting room filled with a variety of activities to entertain children. Some children want to play with blocks (regardless of age) or read one of my Animal Planet books, while other children cannot wait to get their hands on their parent's iPhone or iPad. Understanding the type of child you have and tailoring an approach to help him develop a healthy relationship with screens, mobile devices, and tablets is essential to his emotional health.

One real challenge is the fact that children are digitally smarter than we are. Emily, a twelve-year-old client, is an Instagram star and has more than 10 million views of the last song she posted. I asked to see it. She quickly replied, "My mom turned off my apps," and then a second later realized, "Wait, I can turn it back on without her knowing."

What I know for sure is that helping our children develop a healthy relationship with screens doesn't actually have to do with screens themselves — it has to do with cultivating honesty, self-control, and attentional abilities. These are the game-changing skills that when grown can be applied across the board — whether that's helping your daughter (like Marisa) turn off the television without a major meltdown or helping your son tell you how he's really feeling. (In chapter 5 we'll discuss attentional abilities and how to help a child focus and learn how to increase his or her self-control.)

TAKE NOTE

SCREEN TIME

Our devices give us instant access to the world, which is both exhilarating and distracting. Since I recently lived through the Montecito mudslide (it was only two miles away from where I live), I became somewhat glued to the screen. It was unhealthy for me, so I took a "screen detox" for three days and felt instant relief from stress. Of course, this approach doesn't work for everyone, but for me at that time it helped immensely. Here are some ideas from screen-time experts to help set you on an emotionally healthy course:

- **Do a digital detox.** Take a day and go hiking with your children without using any screens (but do take a mobile, just in case). *Reset Your Child's Brain* by Victoria Dunckley shares a screen-detox approach to resetting your child's brain.

- **Use a bucket.** Mentor your children by implementing a "bucket rule," in which all phones and tablets go into a bucket at dinnertime so that real conversation and connection can happen.

> • **Set family screen rules.** Create a set of media-healthy rules for your family that you can abide by. *Screenwise* by Devorah Heitner is an excellent resource for helping you mentor your children in their use of digital devices.

Up Next

Now that we have a big-picture understanding of emotional health, we're ready to dive into the nitty-gritty. In chapter 3, I introduce the seven life-changing ideas that can help children get unstuck from patterns and move toward making smarter emotional choices. We will also explore the emotionally healthy mindset, so that we not only provide our children new ideas but cultivate their capacity to be flexible and responsive, versus reactive and rigid. I believe it's all possible for your child, so let's continue together on this journey of positive emotional health.

Part Two

MINDSET

Chapter Three

IDEAS

The basic premise that children must learn about emotions is that all feelings are okay to have; however, only some reactions are okay.

DANIEL GOLEMAN

When I was a child I would climb the weeping willow in my backyard. It was a majestic tree with many limbs. I remember feeling on top of the world because I could climb up till I was higher than my house. When my father came outside looking for me, he never looked up. So the tree became my refuge, a place of calm and quiet.

Looking back, I realize that this is one of my earliest memories of regulating my emotions. When my parents argued (usually over household chores like grocery shopping), I would go outside and literally climb a tree.

Children typically don't have to climb trees anymore to find peace. That's the good news. But boys and girls still need to learn the skill of balance, which is at the heart of emotional health. When a child is angry, fearful, scared, or nervous, he is off-balance. When a child isolates herself and shuts down emotionally, she is off-balance. Getting off-balance is a normal part of being human, but learning how to bring oneself back into balance is at the core of emotional health.

Since many of my lessons (and probably yours, too) were hard earned, I feel very hopeful that children can benefit from what we now know — said simply, they don't need to go through the same unnecessary bumps in the road. Boys and girls can learn at an early age how emotions work and what to do to bring themselves back into balance sooner rather than later. In this chapter, I share:

- *Ideas.* Some life-changing ideas, which, when children learn them, can help them start mastering their emotions and come back into balance sooner.
- *Mindset.* We all know that mindset matters, but what is an emotionally healthy mindset? And how can we nurture this mindset in our children?

Of course, even though my focus is on helping you raise emotionally healthy children, the ideas and tools in this chapter work just as well for adults. What makes them healthy makes us healthy, too.

The Skill of Balance

To put it as simply as possible, balance is crucial for every aspect of your child's functioning.
DANIEL SIEGEL AND TINA PAYNE BRYSON

Molly, ten years old and in fifth grade, got out of balance when she was playing with her best friend, Jade. Two other girls, Sara and Edna, approached them and invited only Molly to a playdate on the weekend. Molly was surprised and saw that after the girls left, Jade had tears running down her face.

Of course, Molly was happy to be invited to hang out but felt terrible for her best friend, Jade. She told her, "That wasn't very nice of them," and Jade agreed. But then Molly got off-balance even more by trying to fix Jade's hurt and not doing what she wanted to do — she wanted to play with different friends at recess but instead played only with Jade daily to make her feel better.

Since I'm a visual learner, I want to share what it looks like when your child is off-balance and also when he or she's moving in the right direction:

Off-Balance	Healthy Balance (in the process of learning)	Optimum Balance
• is reactive • isolates self • shuts down (doesn't say a thing) • has excessive or dramatic outbursts, such as crying, screaming, slamming doors, and saying mean things • hurts self or others • has physical complaints (regular headaches and stomachaches)	• is learning to respond • gets triggered but is learning how to display self-control (over body and mind) and make smarter choices • feels all emotions and doesn't ignore any of them, but seeks to express them constructively (much of the time)	• is responsive • has learned to calm and center self even when challenged • makes choices from a calmer place, most of the time • creates emotionally healthy habits, such as exercising, talking to friends, journal writing, and volunteering *continued on next page*

continued on next page

Off-Balance	Healthy Balance (in the process of learning)	Optimum Balance
• needs to learn the skill of balance (ideas and tools)	• has a few emotional tools he or she uses daily (deep breaths, music, yoga poses, gratitude list) • continues to have regular emotional upsets but is learning from them	• has emotional tools he or she uses daily • has an emotionally healthy mindset (more in this chapter) • has periodic emotional upsets but comes back to balance easily (much of the time)

Although I'm primarily focused on helping your child get his mind and emotions back into balance, of course his body needs to come back into balance, too. I remember being a nervous test taker in elementary school and getting full-body hives during standardized testing (guess how I still feel about them). But most often when a healthy child's mind and emotions return to a calmer, more balanced state, her body follows suit.

Coming Back into Balance

We can be sure that the greatest hope for maintaining equilibrium in the face of any situation rests within ourselves.

FRANCIS J. BRACELAND

Coming back into balance happens differently for every child, but there are tools that can help any parent or teacher. For example,

I am a big fan of deep breaths, especially when a child has gotten off-balance in a challenging direction.

Joshua is angry and wants to hit someone, but he's at school and doesn't know what to do. He could take five deep breaths in through his nose and out through his mouth, no matter where he is.

Or perhaps he'd rather put one hand on his heart to reconnect with his body and slow down. He could also say, "Everything is okay," and by his positive self-talk could calm himself. The point is that children like Joshua need some sort of a tool or strategy to apply when they're off-balance, and their breath is with them wherever they go. Unlike the ubiquitous fidget spinners used for hyperactivity, these tools are invisible.

Many of the children I've seen say, "Deep breaths don't work," and that simply means they're not doing it correctly or that they dislike this approach. Either way, there are other strategies that can help a child stop and calm himself, such as:

- closing his eyes
- walking away (maybe taking a bathroom break and splashing water on his face)
- taking child's pose (a yoga pose that is easy to do, if permitted)

The point is to interrupt the anger, frustration, and fast-moving energy so your child can slow down and calm before making a not-so-smart choice. There is no one right method for bringing a child back into balance; you can work with your child to see what tools fit best with his or her temperament. In the next chapter I go into detail about different methods that have worked with children around the world. Coming back into balance isn't merely a matter of good luck or great genes (although they help) but simply a skill to be learned.

TAKE NOTE

EMOTIONAL COACHING

Children will only accept our coaching when we have formed a good connection with them, which makes perfect sense. Along with forging a strong connection with our children, we also need to co-regulate with them before they can master their emotions. Here are some key ideas to remember when coaching your child:

- **Connection.** Connection is the ability to create a healthy relationship with your child based on authenticity, cognitive empathy, and clear communication. Children must feel like their feelings matter, that you appreciate their perspective (although you may not agree with them) and want them to be happy. Said simply, they must feel you're on their emotional team versus against them.

  Years ago, my friend's son told me that when his father spoke to him, he simply got "the talk" because there was no empathy, no validating of emotions, just lecturing. Children don't learn from lecturing (neither do we); they just hear "blah, blah, blah." But when you tell them you hear them and you validate what they're experiencing, you can make a genuine connection with them.

- **Emotional coaching.** Emotional coaching consists of mentoring children about what emotions are, how they work, and what they can do to constructively express them. It involves ideas and tools — and practice. But the best emotional coach is the one who models positive emotional health and not only talks the talk but walks the walk. By no means am I saying that we need to be perfect. None of us are, but we must do our part to live honest, healthy, and authentic lives, and when we make mistakes, we apologize and teach our children how to course-correct without shame or guilt.

- ***Co-regulation.*** Regulating your child's emotions along with them until they can start regulating their emotions alone is called co-regulation. You're in balance, or you know how to bring yourself back into balance, and you allow your children to lean on you for support. For example, your son was crying because he wasn't invited to a birthday party, and then he climbed into your bed. You did what most parents would do — you hugged him, rubbed his back, and said, "It's going to be okay." This is co-regulation, which helps him regain his balance and learn to self-soothe, which is necessary for self-regulation.

The Basics of Emotions

Feelings come and go like clouds in a windy sky. Conscious breathing is my anchor.

THICH NHAT HANH

One thing I learned from traveling around the world and sitting at the feet of happiness teachers is that emotions work in a certain way. When I was surrounded by a band of monkeys on a mountain in India I was terrified, and when I was welcomed with open arms in London by new friends I was delighted. Emotions are par for the course in our everyday lives, but how we handle these ups and downs is informed by our understanding of what emotions are and how they work.

In this section we'll discuss how to help children get a handle on how emotions work, and what they can do to move themselves in a healthier direction. The ideas presented may sound simple, but

I have found that if you don't get the small stuff correct, it's harder to move up to the bigger things. If Frankie doesn't learn to handle his frustration over sharing his toys with his sister, for example, he may miss out on the enjoyment of having someone to play with.

My goal is to provide you with simple yet life-changing ideas to nurture your child's emotional health, and ultimately, happier life experiences. Of course, they're not magic, but they are the seeds of emotional mastery, which when learned young can put a child on a positive trajectory. The seven ideas that children need to learn are:

- Emotions are temporary.
- Inside of you (at the center) is joy, your natural state.
- There are different types of emotions.
- Mixed emotions are common.
- All emotions are useful; they are simply sending you signs about what's happening inside of you.
- You can learn how to increase certain emotions (the helpful ones) and reduce other emotions (the challenging ones) with practice.
- No one can do it for you.

Each idea needs to be shared at your child's appropriate age level, and then deepened over time. Let me expand on those ideas here.

1. *Emotions are temporary.* No matter what emotion you're experiencing — happiness or anger — it's temporary. Boys and girls, especially those who suffer from sadness, often mistakenly think that emotions are permanent. They think the big, dark cloud over their heads will never leave, but that's not true. By thinking a new thought, they can often feel a new feeling, and the clouds will pass (most of the time).

"This too shall pass" is a motto used by many adults to remind themselves of the temporary nature of emotions and can be helpful on a hard day. Children can also create their own mottos such as, "Big feelings come, and big feelings go."

2. *Inside of you (at the center) is joy, your natural state.* At the center of our being is goodness, which equates to pure positive energy or joy. This is your child's natural state. But his or her challenging feelings — anger, sadness, worry, panic, frustration, disappointment, and jealousy — can cloud that natural state. But if your child learns to let these challenging emotions pass by like clouds, the inner sun (goodness) can shine again.

   Learning how to let feelings — especially tricky feelings like anger — come and go takes practice. But using a tool like mindful breathing, which Thich Nhat Hanh calls his "anchor," can help a child slow down and let the big emotions pass by as he breathes through these challenging moments.

3. *There are different types of emotions.* Children experience a full range of emotions, from misery to happiness, but they don't necessarily understand the different types of emotions. Some types are: fast and slow, big and small, challenging and easy, and positive and negative. For example, anger is a fast emotion and also often feels very big and can be hard to tame without training (like a big lion). But when a child realizes she is bigger than her anger, she can muster her courage and learn how to let her anger go without making not-so-smart choices.

   Helping children learn about the different types

of emotions and how to connect with them in a healthy way happens over time. When reflecting on a big feeling in a calm moment, some conversation starters may be: "Did that emotion feel bigger than you? Did it happen quickly? Did you feel it when it was small? If so, where in your body did you feel it?" (In chapter 4 I provide more detailed information on strategies to help with various emotions.)

4. *Mixed emotions are common.* Children often feel more than one emotion at the same time, such as when a pet passes away. Ten-year-old Helene had known Moby, her black Labrador retriever, her whole life and was incredibly sad when she died. But Helene also felt re-lief that Moby wasn't suffering anymore in her old age. Helping children name their emotions, especially when they're mixed and complicated, is the first step toward helping them constructively express them.

Once Helene named her feelings as "sadness" and "relief," she could begin letting those feelings move through her. She painted a special rock for Moby and laid it on her grave, which helped Helene feel a little better.

5. *All emotions are useful.* Your emotions are simply sending you signals about what's happening inside of you, so every emotion is useful, whether it feels chal-lenging, like disappointment, or easier, like excite-ment. Learning how to spot emotions when they're small (like a little frustration before it becomes a volcano-size anger) will help you constructively ex-press it. No emotion needs to be wasted — every-thing can be used as a stepping-stone to your next best feeling.

Helping children realize that emotions are neither good nor bad but simply signals is essential to their positive emotional development. Conversation starters around this subject include talking about street signals (stop signs, police sirens, and traffic lights: red, yellow, and green). What do they mean? Are emotions like anger, joy, sadness, or silliness sending signals, too?

6. *You can learn how to increase certain emotions (the helpful ones) and reduce other emotions (the challenging ones) with practice.* Once children begin to realize that they can turn up the volume on certain emotions and lower the volume on others, the world is their oyster. There is nothing they cannot accomplish. The first step is giving children the ideas, and then the tools (more on this in chapter 4), while nurturing inner qualities of positive emotional health (chapter 5).

Being thankful is not just reserved for Thanksgiving Day. Gratitude is an emotion that moves children in a positive direction, no matter what. Every night, Hayyam makes a gratitude list as he lies in bed reflecting on his day. He's been thankful for everything from jelly beans to a new karate teacher, and feeling this appreciation, instead of focusing on what he doesn't have, helps him realize how good things really are in his life.

7. *No one can do it for you.* Children must learn to take responsibility for their emotional lives and realize that they're the captains of their emotional ships. They can learn to steer toward calmer waves and

through the rough ones with more ease. Just like ship captains, they must get training on how to navigate the "high seas of emotions" of anger, rejection, embarrassment, hurt, and feeling left out, for example. But with ideas, tools, and practice, children can become fully themselves in an authentic, meaningful way.

Ernie's Emotions

Ernie was in trouble weekly for getting into conflict on the playground. His parents, Margarita and Luis, promised to get him some professional assistance. Meeting with Ernie, I found he simply didn't know how to identify his emotions or express them constructively. Of course, this isn't rocket science, but in helping Ernie I started with the basics of emotions such as:

- Emotions are temporary.
- You're in charge (no one can do it for you).
- You can learn how to feel good and release challenging emotions in better ways.

Ernie was genuinely surprised to learn he was in charge and could do things differently. I asked, "Did you know you have a choice when you're angry?" He shook his head no. Helping children realize they have a choice empowers them and helps them see they can do things differently — in a way that's good for them and others.

Next, I gave Ernie an "Emotional Faces Sheet," which we filled out together, to help him begin to identify emotions. The sheet has empty faces and feeling names below each face. Ernie drew what each emotion looked like to him. I helped by making the expressions (with my face) to illustrate each emotion, such as sadness, anger, silliness, love, disappointment, frustration, and happiness. To my surprise, Ernie loved doing this exercise. Just for equality's sake, I then filled out the same form and let Ernie make the same faces so he could feel what those emotions felt like in his body, too.

Being able to name emotions is always the starting point in emotional learning and self-regulation. If your child doesn't know he's sad, how can he constructively express it? But once he names and accepts "I'm feeling sad," he can then apply a coping skill to release that emotion and let it pass by like a cloud on a rainy day. He is no longer fooled into thinking that the emotion will last forever.

Once Ernie started to identify his emotions when they were pebble-size versus Eiffel Tower–size, we worked on adding tools to his emotional toolbox. Ernie even drew some literal tools, including a sledgehammer, a shovel, and a pickax, to symbolize what he was learning. As any skilled elementary school teacher knows, the more concrete the example the better.

Some of Ernie's early tools included walking away, using positive self-talk (mottos to talk him down when he grew frustrated), and doing breathing exercises. Interestingly, Ernie took to the deep breaths and said that "blowing out birthday candles" (a breathing exercise) really helped him calm down.

Children like Ernie who traditionally have been very emotionally reactive can learn to do things differently. They can learn to slow down using mindfulness exercises (more on this in chapter 5), stop, and make a new, smarter choice. But they cannot do it alone — they need a parent, teacher, or mentor who sees their inherent goodness and can coach them toward positive emotional health.

TAKE NOTE

LEARNING CAN BE FUN!

Children love things that are fun, especially when they're dealing with emotions, which can be tricky for them to express in words. Some of the tools I've found helpful in early-learning classrooms and at home are:

- *Kimochis* (www.kimochis.com) sells "feeling bags," to help children start to identify and label their varied feelings. I have used the bag with young children, and they tell me about the moments when they've felt left out, embarrassed, cranky, brave, hopeful, and more. Kimochis also offers a curriculum for early education (preschool, kindergarten) to help children begin to name and regulate their feelings. Their Lovey Dove is a large dove that can hold the feeling toys inside her pouch.

- *Feelings Playing Cards* by Jim Borgman. This is a normal deck of fifty-two cards, except with feeling words on them. They can also be used as a regular deck of cards.

One parent told me about a "feelings book" he created for his daughter, Delilah, which became her favorite book. He took photos of her face showing different emotions, printed them out, and then cut out the images, with the feeling name below each face. She took this book with her everywhere.

Mindset Matters

I think anything is possible if you have the mindset and the will and desire to do it and put the time in.

ROGER CLEMENS

Merriam-Webster defines *mindset* as "a mental attitude or inclination," while the Oxford Living Dictionaries calls it "the established set of attitudes held by someone." The word *mindset* goes back to 1920, when it was first used by educators to describe someone's mental habits gleaned from life experience — *mind* (noun) and *set* (verb). Mindsets are formed by what we learn and how we experience the world.

Fast-forward to 2006, when Carol Dweck revolutionized the concept of mindset with her book *Mindset: The New Psychology of Success*, helping to bring the idea of a growth mindset into a global discussion. She writes that "in a growth mindset, people believe their most basic abilities can be developed through dedication and hard work — brains and talent are just the starting point." What I love about a growth mindset is that it empowers children and inspires optimism, because nothing is fixed. A child can learn from her mistakes, pick herself back up again, and then try again — whether her goal is to become a junior lifeguard or to feel less nervous while test-taking.

Emotionally healthier children have a growth mindset, which helps them learn from their mistakes. They also realize that everything can be used as fodder for their best life, which helps soften disappointments, failures, and rejection. The failed test is simply signaling you may have to study more or in a different way. When children recognize that emotions are simply signals to what's happening inside them they can take note, learn from the situation, and move forward, ready to create a better feeling, even if it's a tough day.

Coaching children to see themselves as capable and able to learn from their experiences helps them to adopt a growth mindset as well as become emotionally healthier. Though the mindset of emotional health reaches beyond the growth mindset, it is a pivotal idea because every child needs to know they can learn, change, and grow from their experiences and efforts.

The Mindset of Emotional Health

We create most of our suffering, so it should be logical that we also have the ability to create more joy. It simply depends on the attitudes, the perspectives, and the reactions we bring to situations and to our relationships with other people.
HIS HOLINESS THE FOURTEENTH DALAI LAMA

Changing your mind is changing your mindset. Every child's mindset is a work in progress, but early on they begin to form beliefs about their emotions and whether they can express them or need to run from them at all costs.

The emotionally healthy mindset, which begins with learning the seven ideas discussed earlier in this chapter, is something we can cultivate in our children over time. Complementing what children need to know (those earlier ideas) are certain *characteristics* of the emotionally healthy mindset, which I share here:

THE EMOTIONALLY HEALTHY MINDSET

- sees emotions as neither positive (+) nor negative (-)
- stays in the present moment
- faces the present with courage (strength, grit, inner confidence)
- seeks positive choices (for self and others)
- allows emotions to come and go without clinging (attachment) or avoiding them (aversion)
- uses emotions as a guide toward well-being

The emotionally healthy mindset isn't all rainbows and uni-corns, but a child with this mindset simply faces any emotion with courage and lets it move through her. Jenny is thrilled she's going to zoo camp this summer, and Marcus is saddened that his best friend, Jake, is moving to another state. Jenny and Marcus are experiencing different feelings, but they aren't ignoring them, suppressing them, or having knee-jerk reactions to them. They're facing their emotions and expressing them constructively.

Mindset in the Making

While children are learning to see their world more skillfully and starting to steer their emotional ships toward well-being, they're also forming a healthier mindset. There are also certain qualities, which we can help them develop, that can contribute mightily to the formation of this mentality (see the following boxed section).

THE EMOTIONALLY HEALTHY MINDSET

open-minded
adaptable
willing to learn and change*
flexible*
responsive*
positive self-perception*
connected
values goodness (compassion, kindness, forgiveness)

SKILLS LEARNED WHILE FORMING THIS MINDSET

communication*
relational

emotional regulation (skill of balance)*
ability to handle discomfort*
resilience*
cognitive control*
impulse control*
mindfulness (the skill of insight)

Although all the attributes of the emotionally healthy mindset are important, the starred ones indicate essential attributes. An emotionally healthier child is learning how to respond versus react, communicate her emotions, focus her mind (cognitive control), and regulate her emotions, which widens her ability to handle discomfort.

Stages of Emotional Health

Cultivating the mindset of emotional health happens in stages, but some of the accelerators are mindfulness strategies, emotional mentors, and emotional education. In this chapter, we began to discuss in earnest what children need to know — and how to help them learn those foundational ideas. Coming up, we'll delve more deeply into strategies for helping our children slow down and make smarter choices.

But before we do, let's look at a visual of the emotionally healthy mindset and where it comes from.

An Emotionally Unhealthy Child Is:	Becoming Emotionally Healthier	An Emotionally Healthy Child Is:
Reactive	～～～➔	Responsive
Rigid		Flexible
Careless		Mindful
Ignores feelings	～～～➔	Shares feelings
Crushed easily		Resilient
Disconnected		Connected
Insecure	～～～➔	Secure

The line from an emotionally unhealthy to an emotionally healthy mindset is not a straight line but clearly a squiggle. This represents a child's process of learning how to stop, calm, self-soothe, identify emotions, apply antidotes, and turn up the volume on helpful emotions. One of the reasons I love teaching children and parents about emotions is that I have had one of those squiggly lives, which taught me about pain and suffering as well as how to become healthier and happier.

On the path to becoming healthier and happier I've also been enormously helped by teachers and mentors. They were able to see in me what I couldn't see in myself in those emotional moments, and they helped me through the inevitable squiggles of life, which we do with our children every day.

Cultivating Mindset in Children

You have to apply yourself each day to becoming a little better. By becoming a little better each and every day, over a period of time, you will become a lot better.

JOHN WOODEN

Last week I watched the documentary *Jane*, about Jane Goodall and her journey from her home in the United Kingdom to Gombe Stream National Park in Tanzania to study chimpanzees. In it Jane states, "It was my mother that gave me self-esteem." Her mom supported her interest in animals, which enlivened her dream of studying animals in the wild.

It is not only what we say but the messages we send our children that help them form their self-perception and mindset. Of course, mindsets can change, but it's those early memories and experiences that are so potent, such as Jane's father giving her a stuffed gorilla, which to this day sits on her dresser in London. What seemed like a small gift became a symbol of something far greater for Jane.

The mindset of emotional health is not only supported by having loving and supportive parents; it is formed by learning particular ideas, and then trying them out and gaining insight:

Mindset of Emotional Health

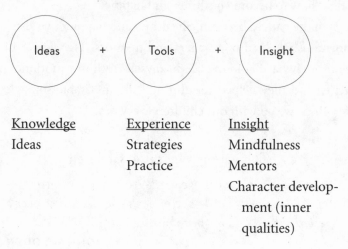

| Ideas | + | Tools | + | Insight |

Knowledge	Experience	Insight
Ideas	Strategies	Mindfulness
	Practice	Mentors
		Character development (inner qualities)

Coaching children to understand what emotions are and how they work is considered knowledge acquisition, which began in this chapter but continues throughout this book. Boys and girls who can learn about their emotions and then apply a strategy to express them constructively are on the way toward forming an emotionally healthy mindset.

Coupling knowledge with tools isn't the whole picture, though. The emotionally healthy mindset also consists of developing positive inner qualities, which I term *character*. It's the mindset of wanting to do good and not to hurt other beings. Though this may seem obvious, forgiveness, kindness, compassion, and empathy don't come naturally to every child, but with our help, they can learn those skills so they can live their healthiest and happiest lives.

Coming Up

Up next, I share practical tools and methods to help your children calm, center, and make smarter choices, the tools of emotional health. While it's not an exhaustive list, these strategies are a solid start to emotionally coach your children on managing their emotions and helping them become the captains of their fate.

Chapter Four

TOOLS

A good teacher isn't someone who gives the answers out to their kids but is understanding of needs and challenges and gives tools to help other people succeed.

JUSTIN TRUDEAU

Sometimes we're so busy we forget to see who our children really are and what they need at each stage, and that's why seeking support from others can be so life changing. Other times we are too close to the situation to see the whole picture and remember what we need to do. This is especially true in emotional moments. Tammy told me this about her daughter, Katie: "She's constantly mean and negative. Today when she didn't feel well, her brother asked me how she was — he was being thoughtful. But as soon as Katie came out of the bathroom, she barked at her brother, 'It's none of your business,' and went into her room, slamming the door. This is just one small example of how Katie treats everyone."

Tammy's exhausted, and for good reason. Katie responds very negatively to situations, whether she's being mean to her brother or refusing to do her spelling words. At the tender age of six, Katie is already in a pattern of negativity and quick reactions, and she doesn't yet have the skills to constructively express her challenging emotions.

But Tammy cannot see this right now. She simply says, "I cannot take her mean streak anymore!" Of course, I understand that the demands of parenting are great, which means it's not always easy to see things from your child's perspective.

Helping Tammy see her daughter differently and have more compassion for her is my first order of business. When Tammy sees her daughter not as a "problem child" but as someone who is simply lacking emotional skills, she can muster the energy to be more patient and help her, which is what Katie desperately needs.

In this chapter I share the tools parents and educators can use to help children like Katie come back into balance, find their center, and make smarter choices. Katie is a good example of the emotionally reactive child; these children aren't easy to parent or teach, but they aren't uncommon, either. And to be honest with you, I was an emotionally reactive child, which is why I understand them from the inside out.

Emotional Imbalances: Hot and Cold

Happiness is not a matter of intensity but of balance, order, rhythm, and harmony.

THOMAS MERTON

Some children run "hot" when they get upset, which means they get annoyed, frustrated, and mad easily. They are quick to anger and have quick reactions to their discomfort. Boys and girls who run hot may say mean things like, "You hate me" and "You want me to be miserable." They're speaking from an angry place and perhaps later may apologize. But their anger in that moment is real and overwhelming to them and needs to find expression, which helps children find relief. Other not-so-smart ways children find anger relief include screaming, slamming doors, stomping feet, punching, biting, and throwing things.

Let's remember: Anger is normal and healthy. But the way we respond to anger is what matters, and how we teach our children to do so is essential. All children, especially those who tend to run hot with anger, need constructive ways to release their emotions. Of course, everyone gets angry, but some children — by their nature and patterning — tend to run hotter than others, presenting some distinct parenting challenges.

> Examples of what children running hot might do:
> - sass you back
> - throw a book or other object at you
> - push another kid on the playground
> - scream when told no

Other children tend to run "cold" when they get upset, which means they become sad, depressed, and lonely. They tend to internalize their emotions and withdraw from the outside world. Boys and girls who run cold may say, "Leave me alone" and want to be left in their bedroom to cry. They may feel sad and believe that no one understands them, and therefore they withdraw from their regular activities that previously gave them joy.

Sadness is normal, and it is certainly a healthy response to different life events, but a child who repeatedly runs cold needs to learn ways to find balance again. Of course, there are moments in every child's life that feel particularly challenging, whether her parents are divorcing, someone has died, or she is being bullied, but those are moments in time and don't need to be the permanent weather forecast.

> Examples of what children running cold might do:
> - go into their bedroom to cry alone
> - sulk and pout
> - say, "I'm no good at anything"
> - refuse to go on playdates that previously brought joy

Whether your son or daughter runs hot most of the time, with a short fuse, or cold, with the looming possibility of sinking into a funk, they are getting off-balance, and they need to learn tools to help them rebalance. I do want to be clear here — children with complex problems may need additional support, such as a psychiatrist or physician.

The upcoming tools are meant for the normally functioning (yet emotionally reactive) children who are capable of learning more and doing better. They may not be perfect children, but they are smart and capable of doing things differently — they just haven't yet learned how.

TAKE NOTE

TAKE YOUR OWN TEMPERATURE

What's your temperature? Along with teaching your children new tools to help them regain their emotional balance, it can be helpful to think about your own tendencies:

- Do you run hot or cold?
- What are your triggers?

- How do you regain your balance?
- Did your parents run hot or cold?

Understanding your own tendencies increases your awareness and thus your ability to respond instead of react when you're faced with a situation that usually throws you off-balance. Of course, the more you know about yourself, the better emotional choices you can make and the better you can show your children how to do the same.

Anger: The Hot Child

Holding on to anger is like grasping a hot coal with the intent of throwing it at someone else; you are the one who gets burned.

BUDDHA

A young child can become irate because she got the smallest piece of pizza, while an older child can become annoyed when you ask to see the homework that is due the next day. Boys and girls who run hot can get angry sometimes for the smallest of reasons. Some common childhood triggers, especially for hot-running children, are:

- unfairness
- having no choices (being told, "You must do your homework now.")
- impatience (having to wait in lines)
- being talked down to

Although the young child's pizza slice may not have been the smallest, her perception was that it was. It's a child's perception that spurs him or her to feel frustrated, annoyed, agitated, and ultimately angry. When you help a child who chronically sees the negative side of things shift her perspective to a more positive mindset, you're helping to reduce her anger in the long term, too.

Of course, the biggest challenge with anger is its speed. There are often only a few seconds between when a child feels slighted and when the screaming begins. But if we can lengthen the space between stimulus and response, the child who supposedly got the smallest piece of pizza can take a breath and then respond differently. She can learn to calm herself and respond from that calmer place instead of simply running on automatic.

By bringing the thinking portion of her brain (left side) online sooner, she can stop before reacting and demonstrate some impulse control. While learning how to do this doesn't usually happen overnight, your child can practice becoming more aware of her feelings and learn to slow down instead of making a not-so-smart choice when she's angry.

Catching Anger Cues

Between stimulus and response there is a space. In that space is our power to choose our response. In our response lies our growth and our freedom.

VIKTOR E. FRANKL

Think back to a moment when you got angry and your anger reached epic proportions quickly. What happened? Did you yell? Spank your daughter? Or say something you wish you hadn't? But imagine if you had tuned in to your anger cues when they were small — you noticed your heart beating faster, or you felt red in the face, or something else particular to you. Would your reaction have been different?

When we catch anger when it's small, we are better equipped to cool down and release this fast-moving emotion constructively. The same is true for our children. Our role is to help our hot-running children learn to catch their anger cues, calm and pause, then make a smart choice about how to express their anger. While we certainly don't want our children to suppress their anger, the question is, How can they express it constructively?

One of my clients, ten-year-old Imani, told me that she imagines her anger falling away when she jumps on her trampoline. By the time she finishes her jumping session, her anger does just that — it falls away. Another client, Marigold, called me about her fourth-grade son, Cole. Cole got into trouble at school for threatening a boy, saying, "If you say that again, I'm going to throw a chair at you"; he had the chair in his hands. His teacher brought him to the principal, who called his parents into her office. Of course, everyone felt terrible — Cole, the teacher, the principal, and Cole's parents, who promised to get him counseling. That's where I came into the picture.

I soon realized that Cole simply wasn't catching his anger cues and didn't yet have the emotional tools to stop, calm, and make a smarter choice. As we know by now, those are the three steps a child can use when faced with anger or any other challenging emotion. Below I provide some words you can use with your own child:

1. *Stop* (or pause). This involves the skill of awareness, so you can catch your emotions when they're small and stop yourself from going down the wrong path.

2. *Calm.* If you catch your anger when it's small, you can learn how to calm down and cool down. This involves learning how to soothe yourself and regulate your emotions instead of letting them control you.

3. *Make a smart choice.* I define a smart choice as being a choice that is good for you and good for others. Smart choices with anger include taking a walk, talking to your teacher, and taking some deep breaths. They don't include throwing a chair at someone or saying mean things simply because you're angry.

Since these are simply ideas, I now share some practical tools to be used for each step (stop, calm, and make a smart choice) so that they can come alive with your child. All healthy children can learn how to catch their anger cues and then apply a calming tool to center themselves. Once centered and calm, a child can learn to make a smart choice, even when she's faced with something challenging.

Step One: Stop — The Skill of Self-Awareness

Children who become aware of their increasing frustrations or annoyances when those feelings are still small are more apt to express their anger constructively. The following tools are to help your child who runs hot begin to develop this self-awareness and to catch himself before his frustrations grow into epic anger.

Of course, there are moments when children have already gone into a full-blown meltdown. This is not the time for using these tools. There are many other tools to help your children constructively express their intensity and anger when they've already reached their boiling point.

Tool 1: Volcano

Volcano helps children understand that their bodies are always sending signals about how they're feeling. Like volcanologists watching a volcano, they can learn to spot the physical signs before they erupt in anger.

Use When

- children need to learn body awareness
- they are disconnected from their bodies
- they are missing the little signs of anger

WHY THE TOOL WORKS

- Children learn to connect with their bodies and pick up on its signs.
- Understanding where children feel anger in their body increases their emotional awareness.
- This teaching tool helps a child (or a whole classroom) learn to see his or her own signs of annoyance, frustration, and ultimately, anger.

HOW TO IMPLEMENT

Tell your children this story, and ask them the provided questions afterward. The goal is to help them identify where they feel their anger when it's small and what warning signs they receive when they're starting to get angry.

> *Story:* What is a volcano? A volcano is an eruption in the Earth's surface where molten rock and lava pour out. Volcanologists study volcanoes, especially looking for the signs of when a volcano is about to erupt so they can evacuate the surrounding areas and keep everyone safe. Scientists keep a close eye on the temperature inside the volcano, and if it gets too hot, they see it as a sign that the volcano may erupt. Also, they look at the plates underneath the volcano, and if those shift or move (like an earthquake), this is another sign that a volcano may erupt. Of course, there are more signs, but the important point is that scientists get signals before a volcano erupts, similar to how we get signs from our body before we erupt in anger.

QUESTIONS

- Do you get physical signs when you're getting angry? Does your temperature change? Does your heart beat faster?

- Where do you feel anger in your body? Do you feel it in your face? Stomach? Hands?
- How long do you feel a little anger before it grows big?
- Do you think you can learn to catch these small signs of anger with practice?

Catching anger when it's small, just as the volcanologists do with volcanoes, helps avoid problematic eruptions. There's no problem with getting angry, but we don't want to explode like a volcano. Instead, we want to learn how to let it go in healthy ways and feel better faster. *Does that make sense?*

What You Will Find

Many children have never reflected on where they feel a little anger in their bodies and what their anger warning signs are. By identifying where they feel anger, children become more self-aware and can begin catching it when it's still small. You'll likely be surprised by your child's answers, which can range from feeling anger in their fists to feeling it in their faces.

Tool 2: Anger Buttons

Anger Buttons helps your children identify their anger triggers and gain self-awareness.

Use When

- children don't recognize their anger buttons
- they are unaware of their triggers
- they repeatedly get angry for the same reason

Why the Tool Works

1. Children need assistance spotting their anger triggers.
2. Understanding what gets them angry can help them make better choices.

3. Connecting how they physically feel anger (Tool 1) and mentally experience it (Tool 2) increases their self-awareness.

How to Implement

1. Have your child (or classroom) take out a piece of paper and with a pen or pencil, divide it into two columns with four rows. Direct children to illustrate in each box recent moments when they got angry. They may use words or drawings, depending on their age and inclinations. Jessie, age eleven, made this chart:

My dad makes me sit at the kitchen table to do my homework, and I want to sit on the floor.	My parents take my phone away at 8:00 PM every night, and I still want to text friends.
The amount of homework I have each week.	Having to get up early and go to school.
Having to be nice to my little sister, who always takes my clothes and ruins them.	Going to soccer when I don't want to.
When my mom makes me do homework before anything else.	Being picked last to play volleyball.

Every child has her or his unique list, which may require several sheets of paper. No matter how they choose to do it, the point is to have children identify when they've gotten angry recently — and I encourage you to do the same. You can do this exercise together, with both of you identifying your anger buttons.

2. Once your child has filled at least one page, review
    to see if there are any patterns. For example, Jessie is
    angry when forced to do something and not given a
    choice. This is one of her big anger buttons. Other
    buttons may include being yelled at, being spoken to
    loudly, or being teased in front of other children. (See
    my book *The Energetic Keys to Indigo Kids* for com-
    mon triggers.)

What You Will Find

Children begin to recognize their anger buttons and identify their
patterns. One child I know gets frustrated when she goes into
loud places or crowded locations like the mall, which prompts
her to get emotionally dysregulated and have a meltdown. As your
children learn about their triggers, their emotional awareness increases, and they can often make better choices.

Tool 3: Anger Name

Anger Name helps children label their anger and distance themselves from the feeling.

Use When

-   children have a sense of humor
-   they identify too closely with being angry
-   they need to realize that anger is a temporary feeling

Why the Tool Works

1. Children learn better when they're having fun.
2. Anger isn't who a child is, and helping children

acknowledge their anger as separate from themselves helps them have an emotional aha.

3. Naming anger helps tame it.

How to Implement

Use the following conversation starter, or use your own words to help your children name their anger and begin to recognize it as a temporary visitor and not a permanent guest. "Bruce Banner is the name of the Hulk when he's not angry, when he's just a normal guy working as a physicist. When someone gets angry they may feel like their 'inner Hulk' might come out and show its face, but that's not who they really are. Do you have a name for your anger when it shows up? If not, let's make one. I need an anger name, too; how about Mad Martha?"

What You Will Find

When children can name something, they can let it come and go more easily. By giving anger a name, they no longer associate themselves so closely with their anger and begin to see it as a temporary visitor. Boys and girls also want to have fun, so the more outlandish the name the better. They will use the name on themselves (like Angry Adam), but when your Mad Martha shows up, they'll tell you that, too, so you can show her the door. By the way, my anger name is Monster Moe. She tends to make appearances in traffic jams.

Step Two: Calm

Calming is an essential part of learning how to self-soothe and regulate one's emotions. Once children can begin to calm, they can take a beat (stop and pause) and then make a smarter choice with a calmer mind.

Tool 4: Bubble Breathing

Bubble Breathing helps children reconnect with their inner calm and expand it through conscious breathing.

Use When

- children are feeling frustrated
- they've caught their frustrations when they're small
- you can connect positively to your children and redirect them

Why the Tool Works

1. Breathing calms the body and soothes the mind.
2. Children can use this tool anywhere.
3. Connecting their breath to a familiar idea helps children remember this tool and activate their imagination (redirect themselves).

How to Implement

1. Explain to your children that breathing is with us wherever we go, and we want to learn a certain type of conscious breathing to help us calm.

   You can even refer back to Tool 3, Anger Name. For example, I would explain that mine is Monster Moe, and describe how, when she shows up and I need to calm myself, I often employ Bubble Breathing, especially during traffic jams and when I'm waiting in a long line.

Notice that I didn't say, "I want you to learn Bubble Breathing because you have a problem" but suggested that I needed it and wanted the child's help. This soliciting of help takes the focus off of him and makes it a tool for everyone. With this approach, the results tend to be more positive.

2. I would say, "Can you help me learn Bubble Breathing? I'm reading about how it doesn't take long, and it helps you feel calmer. The instructions say:

    • Take a deep breath in your tummy, and *imagine you're filling up a bubble*. Hold for one second, and then let it out.

    • Take a deep breath, and now *imagine the bubble surrounding your body*. Hold for one second, and then let it out.

    • Take a deep breath, and now *breathe into a bigger bubble that's covering the whole room*. Hold for one second, and then let it out.

    • Take yet another deep breath, and now *breathe into an even bigger bubble that is bigger than the whole building*. Hold for a second, and then let it out.

    • Take the last deep breath, and *imagine the bubble getting big enough to cover the whole block*. Hold for a second, and then let it out."

3. Ask your children: *How did that feel?* Begin a conversation about breathing and how they can use this tool anywhere to calm down and feel more relaxed. You might even suggest that they draw bubbles in their notebook as a good visual reminder to relax in the classroom and to take five deep bubble breaths. Every

night when your children are lying in bed and getting relaxed, do a few rounds of Bubble Breathing together, and remind them that they can use it anytime.

We are aiming to rewire the brain and create a new, calmer pathway for when your child starts getting hot. He can spot the small signs of impending anger or frustration and say to himself, "I can do Bubble Breathing now and feel calmer." This becomes a default for your child only with practice and is also part of teaching his left brain to come online sooner, especially when his right brain (impulsive reactions, overwhelming emotions) has been running the show.

What You Will Find

By using Bubble Breathing and suggesting to each other to use it, you develop a new language in your household for calming. You'll find many different moments when you can practice Bubble Breathing, perhaps on the car ride home from school or when standing in line at the post office. There isn't an inappropriate place to do Bubble Breathing since it simply helps you calm, find your center, and regain some balance before the volcano erupts.

Tool 5: Hand on Heart

Hand on Heart helps children reconnect with their bodies and to calm before challenging emotions escalate.

Use When

- children need to learn how to self-soothe
- they're resistant to breathing exercises
- they are kinesthetic learners (physically focused and attuned to touch)

Why the Tool Works

1. Self-soothing is helped by physical touch (hugging, patting one's back, rubbing one's arm).
2. Children can use this tool anywhere.
3. Giving a child something to do when he or she is getting frustrated and annoyed helps defuse the situation.

How to Implement

This tool is as simple as it sounds. Ask your children to place their hand on their heart and take ten deep breaths. They can do this either lying down or in another relaxed position.

The "magic" comes because your children get conditioned in moments of relaxation and relate calmness to placing their hand on their heart. This means that in moments of anger, stress, worry, or other uncomfortable emotions this tool can bring them back to a calmer place, especially with deep breaths.

What You Will Find

I love this simple technique because children can be sitting in math class and starting to get anxious, but once they place their hands on their hearts and take some deep breaths, they can feel calmer. Coming back into balance happens more quickly when you find your center and slow down enough to feel your heart beat. I've even taught children to place their hand on their heart and tap their chest, saying, "It's going to be okay," and this is the beginning of true self-soothing. Instead of needing Mom to pat their back, they can learn to pat themselves to feel better.

Let's remember: This tool needs regular practice and modeling to help a child begin to connect Hand on Heart with being calm. Sometimes when I'm in traffic with a carload of little ones, I place my hand on my heart and take a deep breath. Then I ask everyone to help me and place a hand on their hearts, too — and happily, they all do.

Tool 6: Wheel of Feel

The Wheel of Feel helps children realize that they can change what they think about and thus change how they feel in any moment. This is like changing the station on a radio dial, except it's changing your thoughts and tuning in to something better.

USE WHEN

- children are getting angry over "little things"
- they lack cognitive control
- they are able to see things differently but still remain stuck

WHY THE TOOL WORKS

1. Children need a simple tool to reset their emotions.
2. They can get unstuck with a tool.
3. Small changes are possible, while big feeling changes aren't fast or easy.

HOW TO IMPLEMENT

The Wheel of Feel starts where children are and helps them move to a better feeling. Simply ask your children to:

- take out a regular piece of paper
- draw a large circle
- divide it into eight sections, like a pizza pie

Next they'll create their own Wheel of Feel. Instruct them like this:

- In the first section write how you're feeling in the moment. For example, you may write, "I'm angry I have to go to school."
- In the next section, write a better feeling thought like, "I will see my friends at school" and keep going around the wheel with each section.

By the time your child completes the Wheel of Feel she will feel a bit better and begin to realize that she can think a new thought — and then feel a new feeling. Most children need help moving from their stuck thoughts to something that feels a little better. Little by little they'll begin to move, and they can employ this technique whenever they need to feel better.

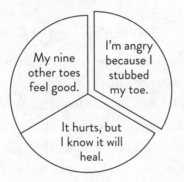

This is only a three-part wheel, but it shows the process. Each section helps your child find a slightly better-feeling thought, which will improve her mood. In this three-slice sample I started with "I'm angry because I stubbed my toe" and moved to something that's a bit better: "It hurts, but I know it will heal" and then to something even just a bit more positive: "My nine other toes feel good," so you see how the process works.

Children need our help changing their thoughts and finding

relief, especially when they feel stuck and angry. Finding a better feeling — even if it's only a little better — means there is movement in a more positive, constructive direction, which is what we want to teach our children they're capable of.

What You Will Find

Children like to feel good and will use the Wheel of Feel when they have challenging emotions such as anger. With practice, they'll learn how to find a better-feeling thought and experience some anger relief as they move in a healthier direction. Chances are they'll also recommend that you complete a Wheel of Feel when you're getting angry, which isn't such a bad idea!

Step Three: Make Smart Choice

Learning how to make smart choices takes time. Being able to make good decisions is a mark of bringing the left brain online sooner and employing a more integrated approach to life. Your child isn't all thinking or all feeling but is learning to find a balance between the two and to understand what's good for him and others. Of course, our focus with this step is making smart choices when children are feeling emotionally challenged.

Tool 7: Smart Choices Checklist

A Smart Choices Checklist is a list of smart choices that children can use whether they're at home, at school, or with friends.

Use When

- children aren't sure how to express their anger
- they repeatedly make not-so-smart choices

- they need to identify constructive outlets for anger relief

WHY THE TOOL WORKS

1. Children create their own checklist, which empowers them.
2. They can make it visible (so they don't forget).
3. Children gain clarity on what smart choices are available to them.

HOW TO IMPLEMENT

Creating a Smart Choices Checklist can be a creative endeavor with your child or classroom. It consists of:

- identifying smart choices when your child begins to feel some frustration, annoyance, or a little anger
- defining smart choices as being good for your child and good for others, and offering some examples. For example, you could say, "It feels good to scream when you're angry, but that's good for you and not good for others. But if you walk away and splash some water on your face to cool down, that's good for you and good for others. See the difference?"
- making a Smart Choices Checklist with your child and hanging it up in her room, which can help her remember what to do when she's upset

SMART CHOICES CHECKLIST: FOR HOME (SAMPLE FOR SALLY)

1. Take deep breaths (Tool 4).
2. Write in my journal.

3. Eat an apple.
4. Shoot hoops in the driveway.
5. Listen to music.

SMART CHOICES CHECKLIST: FOR SCHOOL
(SAMPLE FOR STEPHEN)

1. Walk away.
2. Talk to my teacher (or friends).
3. Write in my notebook.
4. Say a prayer.
5. Do my Wheel of Feel (Tool 6) or Hand on Heart (Tool 5).

Becoming clear on what a smart choice looks like for yourself, and teaching your children to identify smart choices for home, for school, and for time spent hanging out with friends, helps them immensely. Of course, I don't have a problem with children crying, screaming, and shouting, which certainly may feel good to do, but at times doing so may not be the smartest choice. Alexander, for example, was crying in his fifth-grade class, which helped him release his pent-up emotions but got him teased horribly. Learning how to let his emotions out in a way that honored his feelings and didn't cause him social problems in this case would be the smart choice. In the case of Alex, he began journaling, which released his anger constructively and reduced his in-classroom tears.

WHAT YOU WILL FIND

Children like to identify what helps them feel good, and helpful ways to release their big feelings, especially anger. They also like hanging up their Smart Choices Checklist because when they see it in their rooms it helps them remember that they always have a choice in how they respond to their feelings.

Anger: In the Moment

When angry, count to ten before you speak. If very angry, count to one hundred.

THOMAS JEFFERSON

In the moment of anger, children need your presence to serve as a soothing balm to their blistering anger. Of course, we're not perfect in every moment, but that's not our aim; it is to be a refuge for our children, not to take what they say personally or to add fuel to the fire, which is all too easy to do.

But if we can learn how to calm ourselves and be that calming presence for our children, then they can learn to handle their anger constructively. In the moment of anger, your angry children need you to be:

- *Present.* Simply be present. You might say to your child, "I'm here for you."
- *Calm.* Children need to know that everything is going to be okay. The anger will pass, and sometimes we just need to be patient and let a little time go by. You might say, "Let the angry clouds pass" or "This too shall pass."
- *Constructive.* Children need an outlet for their anger, whether that is writing in a journal, building a complex Lego project, or talking to a friend. One of my child clients, Marcos, would go jogging when he got angry, which made him feel a world better. Another client, Kimmy, would hit the punching bag in her basement, which immediately lessened her anger. Guiding your children to make a constructive choice when angry is the work.

Patience is an antidote to anger, so if your son or daughter can muster some self-control even when angry and allow the angry clouds to pass, he or she will begin feeling some relief soon. It takes practice to stop oneself when angry, but I've seen young children take deep breaths and patiently wait for their anger to subside.

Children are also helped by having parents or caregivers who are good anger-management role models. They not only tell children what to do but *show* them how to manage their anger. Children who grow up in families that manage their anger smartly tend to do the same. As discussed earlier, their mirror neurons kick in, and they learn by observing what we do and oftentimes mimicking it.

TAKE NOTE

BEHAVIOR PROBLEMS ARE EMOTIONAL IMBALANCES

Seeing your children's behavior while they're running hot and acting out as a signal that they need to regain their balance is the healthiest perspective. Most of the time, children aren't being difficult on purpose — they merely don't have the skills yet to handle their overwhelming and fast-moving emotions.

As parents, teachers, and professionals, our goal is to help our children regain their balance, whether they're running hot or cold, and to help them build their skills so they can handle life's challenges with more ease. We need to help our children also become more comfortable with discomfort and not simply have knee-jerk reactions. We want them to remember that feelings come and go — and that they are bigger than any of their feelings. We teach them that they can handle whatever life presents and emerge stronger, healthier, and ultimately, whole.

Sadness: The Cold Child

The word "happy" would lose its meaning if not balanced by sadness.

CARL JUNG

Children who run cold or have a tendency toward sadness are genetically hardwired for this proclivity and need our assistance. Of course, there is nothing wrong with sadness and feeling blue. But we don't want our boys and girls to unnecessarily suffer and feel sad with no outer reason for their sadness.

Arming children with the tools for understanding what to do when they feel sad empowers them. They don't need to feel like the gray cloud above their head will never move. It will move, but it may take some assistance (in the form of tools) and some patience (as the gray clouds move away).

Hannah, age ten, has a tendency to run cold and become blue, which is alleviated by:

- talking to friends (making healthy connections)
- getting daily exercise
- reading her favorite books
- eating and sleeping well
- staying on a schedule, which moves her out of her ruts

Just recently Hannah's parents got divorced, and we worked together to help her through this change in family dynamics. Although she was relieved that the fighting had ended, and she would find relief in two happier households, she still needed help regaining her balance. Unlike the child who runs hot and acts out, often with unwholesome behavior, children who run cold tend to withdraw (emotionally and/or physically) and tend to isolate themselves.

One of the keys to helping children who tend to run cold is to help them make and keep healthy connections and to buck their tendency to isolate. They also need to develop the ability to identify their emotions, develop healthy coping mechanisms, and ultimately, make smart choices with their feelings.

Again, the three steps to success are:

1. *Stop.* Children need to develop the skill of awareness not only for their hot emotions but also for their cold ones. Helping children pick up their sadness cues and recognize when they need to come back to center requires that they stop and pay attention to what's happening inside them.

2. *Calm (and connect).* Children who run cold need to calm and find their center and connect with others, since often their natural tendency is to withdraw. Helping children who run cold learn how to make healthy connections and keep them is a vital part of our job as parents, teachers, and caregivers. Children also need to develop a healthy connection with themselves (more on this in chapter 5).

3. *Make a smart choice.* Just as we need to help our children make smart choices when they're running hot (acting out), we also need to when they're running cold (holding in).

Children who can master these steps can move in a healthy direction and learn to stay diligent about recognizing their sadness cues and bring themselves back into balance. The tools shared in this section are aimed at helping your child become self-aware and make healthy connections and, ultimately, smart choices.

REAL-LIFE STORY

ELEANOR'S EMOTIONS

Eleanor, age ten, has a history of feeling down in the dumps because of a challenging home life. Her parents are divorced, her dad recently remarried, and she found out she now has a baby brother: Andy, age two. Her new stepmom, Kim, and Andy just came to live with them from Mexico. This change, along with her temperament of running rather cold, was challenging for Eleanor, so we worked together to help her make smart choices even when feeling blue. Some of those choices include:

- reaching out to a friend
- writing in her journal, especially making a list of things she's grateful for
- exercising

Through our work together, Eleanor realized that she's the master of her emotions and can make a smart choice that will help her feel better, even when she's feeling sad.

Step One: Stop — The Skill of Self-Awareness

Children who run cold need to learn how to stop and recognize when they're feeling sad so they can turn their ship around. Of course, there are moments, such as losing a soccer tournament or having to say goodbye to your pet, when feeling sad makes sense. Sadness and grief are natural parts of living and don't need to be fixed or ignored.

But when I refer to sadness in this section, I'm talking about the child who tends toward sadness, no matter what's happening. They go inward and withdraw when feeling upset versus acting out, like more hot-running children. Again, my goal here is to give you tools to teach your children so they can realize they're the captain of their emotional ship and can steer toward calmer, healthier seas anytime they want.

Tool 8: Iceberg

Iceberg is a tool for cultivating body awareness in your children so they can identify where they physically feel their sadness. Once children can pick up on these cues, they become aware and can make a smart choice about what to do to feel better.

Use When

- children need to learn body awareness
- they are disconnected from their bodies
- they are missing the physical signs of their sadness

Why the Tool Works

1. Children experience sadness in their physical bodies.
2. Helping children identify where they feel sadness in their bodies helps them increase their emotional awareness.
3. Using the metaphor of an iceberg, which is familiar to children, helps them realize that many emotions, including sadness, though unseen are felt.

How to Implement

1. Read the following story to your child, beginning with a question about something he or she may know and feel familiar with.

   Story: "What is an iceberg? It is a floating mass of ice, which can be as big as a house or large building. The majority of the iceberg is underwater, so we cannot see it. Scientists study icebergs so they can keep people safe and steer boats in another direction so they don't hit them.

Similar to icebergs, our feelings, including joy, gratitude, frustration, disgust, and sadness, are mostly unseen and inside us. Being sad is often called being blue, the color of an iceberg. Just like the iceberg, which gives signs to scientists, our bodies give us signs to when we're feeling blue."

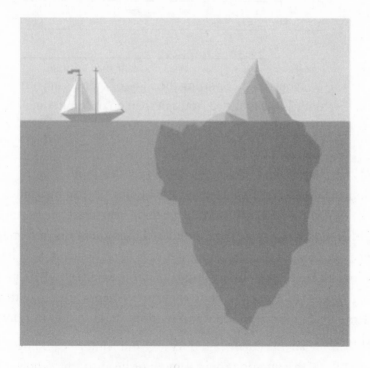

2. Say to your child, "Like an iceberg, which is mostly underwater, our emotions are inside us, and people cannot see them. But if we learn to feel them, and name them when they're small, we can identify them

before they become as big as a house. Where do you sometimes feel sadness in your body? List the places below or on a separate piece of paper."

_____

_____

_____

_____

_____

_____

_____

3.   Tell your child, "Spotting the signs of sadness in your body is the first step. You can then do or think something differently to feel better."

WHAT YOU WILL FIND

Some children are connected to their bodies and can easily identify where they feel sad, such as in their heart, face, or tummy. Other children have never pondered this question and may need quite a bit of help. You might say, "The first step is to become aware of the physical signs of sadness your body is giving you so you can constructively express them without getting tummy aches or headaches and without making not-so-smart choices."

Tool 9: Rearview Mirror

Rearview Mirror helps children stop and get unstuck from looking back at sad experiences. They can learn to move forward wisely by using their power of focus.

Use When

- children repeatedly look at sad things from their past
- they get stuck in sadness
- they aren't yet aware that they can look forward and feel better

Why the Tool Works

1. Children need a simple metaphor for using their focus wisely.
2. They are familiar with cars and see them often.
3. It puts children in the metaphorical driver's seat, and they feel more empowered to make another choice about what to focus on.

How to Implement

1. Start by sitting on the floor or in a chair with your children. Get really comfortable, and let them know they're going to use the power of their imagination for this activity.
2. Lead your children in this activity by using these words or something similar: Imagine you're driving a car, and have fun with it. Actually put your arms on the imaginary wheel and feel yourself in the driver's seat. I have some simple questions now:

    - "Look at your windshield. What is this for? [Answer: To look out of and see forward.]"
    - "Now look at the rearview mirror. How big is this? [Answer: Small.] What is the rearview mirror for? [Answer: To see behind you.]"
    - "Which is bigger, the front windshield or the

rearview mirror? [Answer: The front wind-shield.]"

- "What do you think the universe is telling us by giving us a really big windshield and a small rear-view mirror? [Answer: The world wants you to look forward, not back. You can look back every once in a while, but looking forward is healthier.]"

3. Use this activity as a conversation starter, and share stories from your life about when you looked back, only to feel sad all over again. Looking back isn't al-ways bad, of course, but looking ahead is the healthi-est skill to develop.

What You Will Find

Children like this activity because they enjoy make-believe, and cars are something they're familiar with. The idea that looking ahead is healthier than looking back may be new to them, but it's something children can comprehend. I found it extremely help-ful for young clients, especially middle schoolers, who repeatedly focus on things (worry, obsess, fret) that spiral them into sadness, to learn how to use their awesome power of focus and to look ahead to feeling better.

Step Two: Calm (and Connect)

Children who run cold need to calm and regain their balance (see Tools 4, 5, and 6). They also need to allow their sadness expression in a healthy way, and accept mentoring from emotionally health-ier people, such as parents, teachers, or peers. As we know, the major challenge with cold-running children is their tendency to withdraw and to isolate themselves. This behavior can keep them stuck in sadness. But by making even one healthy connection, a child can move toward better feelings with more ease.

Tool 10: Connect Four

Connect Four helps your children name four connections they can go to when they're feeling sad and low.

USE WHEN

- children repeatedly withdraw from people, places, and things
- they forget the friends in their lives
- you wish your child realized how important relationships are

WHY THE TOOL WORKS

1. Most people are visual learners, and using a visual aid helps immensely.
2. Children can name and claim their connections.
3. There are no wrong answers but simply connections your child can name or look to make.

HOW TO IMPLEMENT

1. Have your child take out a piece of paper and draw a circle, divided into four sections:

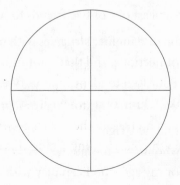

2. In each section of the circle, have your child name a
    healthy connection he has with someone in his life.
    The goal is to name at least four.

Here is an example of a circle, completed by Joshua, age
eleven:

3. Discuss how these four connections, each in its own
    way, helps your child build relationships, which lessens
    his sadness. In Joshua's case, Butter, his golden labra-
    doodle, and Peter, his peer in sixth grade, each have a
    way of helping. You might discuss when to contact and
    connect with each of them and why making, as well as
    keeping, friends is an important part of feeling hap-
    pier. With that said, some children are naturally more
    content alone, which isn't unhealthy, but that child
    does need at least one or two friends to connect with.

Maybe your son or daughter struggles with making friends or
keeping healthy connections, and that's not uncommon. You can
use this Connect Four tool to identify what types of connections
he or she would like. Think of it as a wish list, such as:

•   A new cat named Tiger
•   A friend who makes me laugh
•   A neighbor my age who I can play with

Keep your eyes and ears open for opportunities for your
children to meet that good friend, whether it's at the local arts

after-school program or at a YMCA swimming lesson — an activity that naturally interests your children and where they can meet others is best.

What You Will Find

Children may have one or two people they feel they can talk to, but many struggle with identifying four people or sentient beings (animals included). But the more people you can help your children see as "on their team," the easier it is for them to seek help, especially when they need it. Boys and girls who learn to reach out to their connections instead of withdrawing are healthier and ultimately happier children. Of course, you cannot change your child's personality, especially if she's not a "people person," but you can help her value relationships and develop like-minded friends.

Tool 11: Color It Out

Color It Out helps children get unstuck from their emotions and use a creative outlet to help them come back into balance. Have crayons, markers, colored pencils, or other artwork supplies available to use with your son or daughter.

Use When

- children are stuck in sadness
- they're naturally very creative
- coloring is an activity they enjoy

Why the Tool Works

1. Children of all ages like to color or doodle.
2. Coloring is an evidence-based tool in art therapy that lifts a child's mood.

3. Many children are very sensitive to colors, and using different colors lifts their mood.

How to Implement

1. Connect with your child about how he or she is feeling, and suggest that you color (or do something creative) together to get unstuck from any low feelings. Free coloring sheets can be found at www.growing happykids.com/coloring.
2. Sit with your children, and be a calming presence. This is a moment when you can co-regulate with your children when they're feeling blue. If you're able to stay balanced, then in your presence your children can also move toward balance as they use their creativity to cope with their feelings.

(*Tip:* Don't necessarily talk about emotions in this creative session; simply be the calming and healing presence your child needs. He'll receive your calm and peace just by being near you. Focus on creating together and enjoying these creative endeavors.)

What You Will Find

Creative outlets provide children who tend to run cold with healthy ways to release their sadness and other intense emotions. Although Color It Out is specifically about coloring, it is not the only way. Other creative outlets could be dancing, journaling, gardening, singing, painting, cooking (with assistance), or computer coding. The important thing is to find a healthy outlet for your child where they can find relief from their sadness and discover a new coping mechanism.

Step Three: Make Smart Choices

As we know, helping children make smart choices, however they may be feeling, is an essential part of their emotional education. Of course, some children may need professional assistance, because making a smart choice isn't easy for them until they receive medical or therapeutic intervention. If you wonder if your child may need professional assistance, I lean toward being conservative and suggest getting an expert opinion from a trained professional.

Samantha, age eleven, tends toward feeling blue. She's shy and doesn't have a ton of friends, so when we began working together we made a list of smart choices she could make at home, which lifted her mood:

- Take a bath.
- Jump on a trampoline.
- Read my favorite Harry Potter book.
- Make beaded necklaces, barrettes, and bracelets.
- Have pretzels and orange juice.
- Watch the movie *Elf*, no matter what time of year it is.
- Text my friend, Kate, to get a pick-me-up.

Her mom, Amy, helped her come up with smart choices she could make at school:

- Draw in a sketchbook.
- Go to the bathroom (take a break).
- Read my favorite book in the library.
- Buy an ice cream at lunch.
- Talk to a friend or teacher.

Helping our cold-running children get out of their own way and make healthy connections is part of making smart choices. They need to reach out and accept help as well as realize that sadness isn't permanent but just a temporary feeling. Children can do or think something new to help the clouds pass by.

Beyond Hot and Cold

No one would feel embarrassed for seeking help for a child if they broke their arm — and we really should be equally ready to support a child coping with emotional difficulties.
KATE MIDDLETON

Every child faces emotional challenges at one point or another, but it's how we help that child learn to regain his or her balance that counts. Whether your children run hot or cold or somewhere in between, learning the tools covered in this chapter — especially the Smart Choices Checklist and the Three Steps to Success (stop, calm, make a smart choice) — can help them immediately. Of course, children's emotions are more complex than a simple set of tools, but these tools are a starting point to help children feel capable of handling their big feelings.

Some other challenging emotional experiences many children have are:

- anxiety (worry, nervousness)
- panic attacks
- phobias
- loss
- low self-esteem
- trauma
- obsessive compulsive disorder (OCD)

Genetic factors and environmental stressors also contribute to children experiencing certain emotional difficulties. For example, Aviva suffers from anxiety, and her eleven-year-old daughter, Ellen, already shows sign of nervousness, worry, and a tendency toward feeling anxious about life. Aviva implemented a tool from

Allison Edwards's book, *Why Smart Kids Worry*, called Worry Time; she gives her daughter ten minutes to worry about something, and then the time is up. Worrying time is over. This tool has helped her daughter tremendously.

Finding the resources for you or your child's particular emotional needs is essential. Today there are both trained professionals and plenty of great books that provide clear guidance on how to regain balance.

TAKEAWAY

EMOTIONAL LEARNING

Children need to learn that they are bigger than their emotions and that they can do or think something different to change how they feel. Specifically, if children are feeling a challenging emotion, they can learn to:

- stop
- calm
- make a smart choice

Although these sound simple, they're not necessarily easy. The tools in this chapter are provided to help you teach your children an emotionally healthy way to handle upsetting emotions, whether that is anger, jealousy, sadness, embarrassment, or rejection.

In the sadness section, you will have noticed that I added the word *connect*, so that we had "calm (and connect)." Children who withdraw from others and isolate themselves make things worse for themselves emotionally, and they need to learn how to make healthy connections. Whether they begin with their pet rabbit or their new neighbor, making connections is essential for positive emotional health.

Of course, children's emotions and lives are far more complex than what I can convey in words, but they are enormously helped by ideas, tools, and mentors who can guide them through troubled waters. The goal isn't for our children to have zero challenges but to learn how to sail through bumpy seas and make it to calmer waters.

Up Next

Now that we've given our children the ideas and tools they need to manage their challenging emotions, it's time to shift our focus from challenge to opportunity. Next we will look at planting the seeds of positive emotional health via mindfulness and positive inner qualities so that our children can experience the emotional aha they need to slow down, calm, and make those smarter choices.

Chapter Five

INSIGHT

Mindfulness is the practice of paying attention in a way that creates space for insight.

SHARON SALZBERG

Children who learn tools of mindfulness not only make better emotional choices, but they make better choices overall, in every area of life. As I think back on my childhood, I realize that some of the choices I made were doozies. Whether I was "helping" my mom by putting dish soap in the dishwasher, only later to discover that I had flooded the kitchen with a foot of water and bubbles, or leaving the brownies out where our dog, Muffin, ate them and got sick out her back end (oops), many of these outcomes could have been avoided if I had just slowed down and paid attention.

Choices are what make up our lives. Children who can learn to slow down and use practices of mindfulness can learn to make better choices. Whether that means slowing down enough to read the dishwasher instructions or making more emotionally charged choices such as whether to hit a child on the playground or to walk away, the tools of mindfulness can help.

One of my recent clients, Daisy, age eleven, was feeling insecure and nervous about school, especially her history class. Every morning at around 3:00 AM she would wake up screaming from nightmares, an obvious sign of being out of balance. When I spoke with Daisy, she admitted to "feeling scared" and like she "was going to fail" her history class, but after some coaching she agreed to learn some mindfulness tools and to practice with her mom. I usually expect several days and even weeks for mindfulness strategies to genuinely make a significant difference, but for Daisy the effect was immediate.

By listening to mindfulness audios on Smiling Mind and Headspace, Daisy began relaxing more and focusing on what was important in the moment instead of being scared of the future (or worrying about past mistakes). These mindfulness techniques, along with coaching, helped her turn her emotional boat around and steer toward calmer seas.

In this chapter, I share how mindfulness strategies can help children accelerate the development of their positive emotional health and, ultimately, their wholeness.

Mindfulness

Mindfulness shows us what is happening in our bodies, our emotions, our minds, and in the world. Through mindfulness, we avoid harming ourselves and others.

THICH NHAT HANH

Most of us have heard the word *mindfulness*, which we instinctually recognize as something beneficial for us and our children, but what is it, really? And how can it possibly help, especially in the midst of the daily grind of ensuring that homework is completed, devices are turned off, and drama is kept to a minimum?

One of my clients, Renee, the mother of three boys, noticed a tremendous change in her son, Luis. He began coming home from school wanting to help her and had a positive, calmer presence as compared to his normal "hyped-up and agitated" after-school self. So she asked his teacher, "What is different at school this week?"

Mrs. Moon replied, "We just began using mindfulness exercises every morning in the classroom." Renee was amazed. Although not every child has such a dramatic response, mindfulness exercises really helped Luis calm and connect better.

Mindfulness is proven to help parents and children calm their often overstressed bodies, minds, and spirits. Jon Kabat-Zinn, creator of Mindfulness-Based Stress Reduction (MBSR) programs, explains mindfulness as "paying attention in a particular way: on purpose, in the present moment, and nonjudgmentally." Sounds simple, but not always easy, right? The three aspects of mindfulness emphasized by Kabat-Zinn are:

- paying attention
- being present
- accepting what is (without judgment)

Paying attention is at the core of mindfulness. It's a skill that many children haven't yet developed, especially as it relates to how they feel, what they're thinking, and what others might be thinking of them. Accordingly, many of the strategies in this chapter help children develop the skill of paying attention, which can be applied to how they're feeling and ultimately used to make better choices.

When your child is paying attention fully to what's happening in the now, she cannot be caught in the past or worried about the future. She is in the present moment without getting stuck in mental loops about what just happened or what's going to happen. Being in the present moment, where all your child's power exists, helps her to overcome whatever emotion is happening and let it come as well as go. (Remember the first basic idea of emotions from chapter 3: emotions are temporary.)

Last but not least, Kabat-Zinn emphasizes accepting what is, or seeing things as they are without judging them or labeling them as good or bad. Your son may have gotten a poor grade on his progress report and may be feeling sad about it. This sadness isn't good or bad — it just is. Being with the sadness without judgment and accepting it for what it is — a natural and healthy emotion — is mindfulness. Of course, your child can decide to do or think something different to feel better, but mindfulness allows him to see what's happening without making a judgment about it.

The Age of Mindfulness

Children are uniquely suited to benefit from mindfulness practice. Habits formed early in life will inform behaviors in adulthood, and with mindfulness, we have the opportunity to give our children the habit of being peaceful, kind, and accepting.

DAVID GELLES

Boys and girls who learn how to slow down (mindfulness) versus speed up (mindlessness) are cultivating the capacity to make better choices. They are simply hardwiring their brain optimally earlier in life, which gives them the increased ability to regulate their emotions and demonstrate cognitive control (by choosing their thoughts, for example). Or as *New York Times* reporter David Gelles puts it: "Mindfulness, which promotes skills that are controlled in the prefrontal cortex, like focus and cognitive control, can therefore have a particular impact on the development of skills including self-regulation, judgment and patience during childhood."

In other words, the parts of the brain that are trained by mindful strategies are the same ones that help your child cultivate emotional awareness and balance. Research shows, as we saw with Luis above, that children who participate in mindfulness strategies in the classroom are significantly more likely to display cooperative and pro-social behaviors.

While mindfulness doesn't equal an emotionally healthy child, it does lay the foundation for a child to become aware and then make better choices. Adding practical wisdom (ideas) and tools (practice) to this formula accelerates the creation of the emotionally healthy mindset, which can help a child in her darkest days find the light.

Jeremiah, age eight, learned in the third grade how to take deep breaths to calm down, a very effective mindfulness tool. Before he began using this tool he often did things he later regretted, like pushing his friend on the playground or screaming at his mom during the morning drop-off routine. But with the addition of deep breaths, Jeremiah has been able to calm himself more often and not have as many outbursts.

What mindfulness tools like Jeremiah's deep breaths do is create space between stimulus and response so that children can make smarter choices. When Jeremiah functioned on automatic, he screamed, pushed, and chose to react negatively, which didn't help him or anyone else. But with the addition of mindfulness, he slowed down and began to see that he had more options (especially when he was challenged on the playground) for handling what was often problematic for him.

TAKE NOTE

PRACTICE MINDFULNESS

Children can learn from the get-go how to become more mindful; however, it isn't until age four (in general) that they are able to direct their attention and master their emotions. Every child is different, and there certainly are those who can master these tasks earlier, but a general rule of thumb is that most preschoolers are at the age when mindfulness can be formally taught.

Every child learns from day one how to be in this world. Before she acquires language, she is tuning in to you and receiving impressions or messages. She is picking up on how you're feeling and the tone of your voice. Is your voice rushed or calm? Loud or soft? Every message your child receives is moving her either in the direction of mindfulness or away from it, from a very early age. In other words, your presence is a mighty teacher of mindfulness.

Raising Mindfulness

The attentive, caring, and wise voice of a supportive adult gets internalized and becomes part of the youth's own voice.

NATIONAL RESEARCH COUNCIL

Raising mindful children requires that we become more mindful. This isn't new news, but it does encourage each of us to slow down and reflect on the example we're setting. Of course, each of us — every single one of us — has good days when we're calm and can respond from our sanest self and other moments when we're exhausted and tapped out. This is part of living on this planet and learning how to come back to center faster, even when life throws challenges our way.

So while all the tools in this chapter are for your children, they are also for you. They can help you regain your balance so that you can be the best role model possible. Part of being your best self includes making mistakes, learning how to repair your relationship with your son or daughter, and growing together. Years ago I heard teacher Michael Bernard Beckwith say, "Parenting is a spiritual practice," and I know this is true — so let yourself grow as a person and a parent, especially when it comes to mindfulness.

Raising mindful children is often a group effort. It's about having "all hands on deck" for elevating consciousness — this includes parents, teachers, friends, and family members. It often takes a team of people to help children raise their awareness so they can pay greater attention to their thoughts, feelings, and actions.

Daniel, age eleven, has a tendency to speak loudly and without consideration to others in his family. Though his mom, Cindy, does remind him to use an "inside voice," it's just not something Daniel pays attention to. But just recently his school began teaching mindfulness, and while doing a mindfulness exercise, Daniel had the "emotional aha" that what he says and how he says it tells others about how mindful he is. Later that day, Daniel went home to apologize to his mom for being so loud most of the time.

Becoming more mindful and raising mindful children takes time. A lot of paying attention and practice is involved. While I cannot say that Daniel has never raised his voice again, he did have an insight into mindfulness, and this insight can never be taken away. Once you learn something, you own it, and now it's Daniel's responsibility to respond to his mom and others in a tone and level of voice that is more appropriate.

TAKE NOTE

MINDFULNESS AND FLEXIBILITY

I think of mindfulness as a quality of awareness and the ability to pay attention to what's happening, without judgment. When I stayed at my former Buddhist Center in Redding, Connecticut, I was often asked to sweep the front steps or do the dishes mindfully. There was simply no chore or practice that was considered boring or without merit if done mindfully, the idea being that everything is fodder for your growth — not just the clean dishes but also the dirty ones. Plus, it allows you to practice doing something with your full attention and to cultivate the skill of concentration.

And while mindfulness is a key ingredient in making smart choices, I think of emotional health as having the quality of flexibility (as opposed to rigidity). Attention is needed for mindfulness. Mindfulness is needed to make smart choices, especially when feeling big emotions, but emotional health needs flexibility.

Life is always giving us opportunities to grow, to get off-balance and then regain our balance. I am writing this chapter from my friend's kitchen table in Los Angeles because I've been evacuated from my home due to wildfires. Scarlett, a child client, just emailed me that she's going to PS1 (a local school in Los Angeles) because that school is hosting a Take Your Evacuee to School Day to help children learn flexibility and feel welcome despite being displaced. In sum, adults and children who can remain flexible are better positioned to being emotionally healthy, while those children who are inflexible or rigid have a harder time feeling and being their best emotional selves.

Mindfulness Activities

Wherever you are, be there totally.

ECKHART TOLLE

As we know, both teachers and tools are necessary for positive emotional health and for happier life experiences. We can go fast alone but far together. Learning these strategies can help you become calmer and more apt to have patience with your children as they learn the *how* of positive emotional health.

In this section we will discuss three types of mindfulness activities:

- body awareness
- mind awareness (attention)
- centering

By using the tools in this section, you will be able to help your children slow down and spot feelings in their bodies (body awareness), then use their minds (by paying attention, focusing, concentrating) to make choices that are good for them and others. By teaching centering, you help your children regain their balance, which they need constantly. The mere act of living throws us off-balance, whether it is getting displaced by a wildfire or having a new baby brother. Life is constantly changing, but children who can befriend change will find their balance sooner.

Body Awareness

Our own body is the best health system we have — if we know how to listen to it.

CHRISTIANE NORTHRUP

Helping children become aware of their bodies and pay attention to them can help them learn to calm, self-soothe, and heighten their awareness. Our bodies have many autonomic functions such as breathing, digesting, and even hiccuping, and bringing awareness to them can help us evolve. Years ago, I had a spiritual teacher who claimed that every day she pooped out her troubles and felt better instantly. While I don't have a mindful pooping exercise, it is true that any activity can be fodder for growth and increased mindfulness.

Mindful Breathing

Mindful Breathing is a building block of mindfulness that children can return to over and over to become present and calm.

Use When

- children need to relax
- they're making careless mistakes
- they get agitated easily

Why the Tool Works

1. Mindful Breathing is a scientifically proven way to calm.
2. Breathing exercises are invisible, so children can do them at home, at school, or anywhere they need them.
3. When your child's breath and body calm, the mind can also become calmer, which helps a child make smarter choices.

How to Implement

Mindful Breathing simply means paying attention to your breath. There is no wrong way to pay attention to your breath, but with time children can get better and better (we adults can, too). The mindful breathing activity that I am sharing here is called Five for Five. Follow the steps below to experiment with it, and then teach it to your children.

FIVE FOR FIVE

1. Introduce the activity as a mindful breathing activity, which means you pay attention to your breath.
2. Ask your children to look at their hand (right or left). This exercise is about focusing on your breath, but you use your hand to count to five breaths.
3. You may say something like this: "Let's begin with our hands closed in a fist. This is our hand shut down. But as we take a deep breath in and a deep breath out, we pop one finger out of the fist. The slower we take the breaths, the better. This isn't a race.

    "Let's try our second breath; take a deep breath in, and let it out. Then our second finger goes out of the fist, and we have only three more fingers left. Again, the slower the better, and focus on your breath.

    "Take your third breath in, and let it out. Your third finger comes out.

    "Take your fourth breath in, and let it out. Your fourth finger comes out.

    "Take your fifth breath in, and let it out. Your last finger comes out, and now your whole hand is open. Your palm is flat, and the fist is gone."

    Ask your child: "How do you feel now?"

    When your children are getting agitated or off-balance you might encourage them to do the Five for Five breathing activity. I also suggest having your

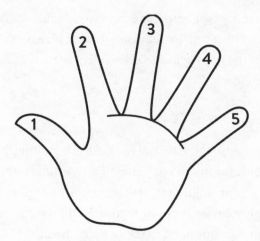

children do three rounds of five breaths, and in one round they focus on the in-breath, on the second round of five breaths they focus on the out-breath, and then in another round they focus on the whole breath — in and out.

The goal of this Five for Five activity is to provide children with an easy way to memorize a simple breathing exercise and to give them a physical memory of it. Sometimes when children are older they don't use the fist but simply touch each finger once. The point is to give them a physical reminder that they're in control of their emotions and that they can use their breath — especially mindful breathing — to calm, center, and let their emotions come and go.

Tip: Don't use Mindful Breathing only to calm your child or to have him regain his balance when he's feeling a challenging emotion. Mindful Breathing is a wonderful way to calm and relax, especially in less volatile times, which helps children make a positive connection with this tool.

What You Will Find

Some children like to do Mindful Breathing when it is connected to a physical activity like blowing on hot soup (see my book *Growing Happy Kids*) or blowing out birthday candles, which is why this Five for Five activity uses the strong physical anchor of the hand to count breaths. Other children are more resistant to breathing activities, which means they may not be ready or may need an alternative way to learn (for example, through mindful breathing audios).

Mindful Seeing

Mindful Seeing teaches your children to be present and to be aware of what's happening around them, especially visually.

Use When

- children aren't mindful of their surroundings
- they can improve their focus and concentration
- they've got a great deal of energy

Why the Tool Works

1. Mindful Seeing is a skill of attention and focus.
2. Children need the direct experience of mindfulness in a way that engages their willingness to explore.
3. Mindfulness can be taught to sharpen all the senses, including sight.

How to Implement

Choose a time when you can go outdoors with your child. Instruct her to walk slowly and carefully. Today's goal is to *see* as many creatures as possible, including things that fly, walk, slither, swim, and move about.

You can ask your child to name the creature when she sees it — for example, I saw a dove and a chipmunk on my morning walk. As you spot the creature, you can have your child:

- name it,
- record it in a notebook,
- photograph it.

The goal is to help children become more aware of what is happening around them and to focus their sense of sight, allowing them to see more. As they increase their ability to concentrate, they become more mindful, and they certainly are in the present moment, too.

What You Will Find

Most children will enjoy getting outdoors and going on a hunt for something like birds, butterflies, or wild animals. When I lived in Asheville, North Carolina, I often saw wild turkeys, deer, and groundhogs in my backyard. They were a joy for me to see. But today's children are often glued to their devices and need a project like this nature expedition to take them away from texting, gaming, and streaming.

Tip: You might ask your child to help you become more mindful and tell her you need her help with an activity called Mindful Seeing. Children often learn better if they think they're helping you or that you're simply having fun. Of course, you can take your children to the zoo or to some special outdoor event, but if possible do this activity in an everyday environment so that they start paying better attention in their daily lives.

Mindful Feeling

Mindful Feeling helps your children pay attention to their physical bodies. The first activity, Jump for Joy, helps your children focus on their heartbeat, which is always there and seldom concentrated on.

Use When

- children are kinesthetic learners
- they have difficulty staying focused on breathing or seeing
- they have an excess of energy

Why the Tools Work

1. Children learn best through direct experience, which these activities provide.
2. Mindfulness can be brought to any activity, including physical ones, especially when it's used to focus the mind.
3. Children begin to realize the cause (jumping jacks) and effect (faster heartbeat) of their actions, which may lead to an emotional aha.

How to Implement

Mindful Feeling consists of two activities, Jumping for Joy and Holding Hands.

Jumping for Joy

Jumping for Joy gives your children the direct experience of physically feeling something and then focusing their minds on this sensation. Again, I recommend doing these activities with your children so that you're learning together (if appropriate and possible).

Here's a sample script:

1. "Complete ten jumping jacks."
2. Afterward, ask your child: "Focus on your heart. Is it beating faster? Can you feel it?"
3. "Complete twenty more jumping jacks. This isn't a competition, so you don't have to rush through them. Take each one nice and slow."
4. Again, ask your child: "Close your eyes and focus on your heartbeat. Where do you feel it? In your chest? Outside your chest? Keep paying attention to your heartbeat, and if your mind wanders, bring it back to your heartbeat. We'll stay focused on noticing our heartbeat for thirty seconds. You can stand or sit, whatever is comfortable. I'll keep the time (use a timer to record thirty seconds)."
5. Say to your child: "Open your eyes. You can do this exercise again later to reconnect with the beating of your heart and the miracle of your body. What did you learn by focusing on your heart beating?"

This first Mindful Feeling activity requires your child be somewhat physically fit, and if that's not possible or advisable, please feel free to adjust accordingly. Instead of completing jumping jacks, he can simply put his hand on his heart and connect with his heartbeat. The idea is to bring focus to the heartbeat, which is happening without your conscious effort, and to bring it into conscious awareness. This helps develop mindfulness.

HOLDING HANDS

The goal of Holding Hands is to help your children to feel physical connection and release stress by holding their own hands. Here's a sample script:

1.   "Examine your hands. Notice them without any judg-
      ment. You may like one hand more than the other.
      That's okay, but appreciate everything about your
      hands and fingers (shape, size, and softness, for ex-
      ample). And don't worry if you need to wash them or
      your nails need trimming; just observe what you see."

2.   "We often think of hand-holding as something we do
      with our parents or someone else. But what if we held
      our own hand? The physical act of holding hands re-
      leases feel-good feelings in our body and helps us feel
      less stressed."

3.   "Put your two hands together and hold your own
      hands. This act helps you calm down and feel your
      fingers touching each other. Close your eyes to ob-
      serve the feelings even more closely. Let's do this for
      twenty seconds and simply feel how holding hands
      feels. If your mind wanders, just bring it back gen-
      tly. Focusing on one thing takes practice. I'll keep the
      time, and let's start now."

4.   "Open your eyes (after twenty timed seconds). You
      can hold your own hands anytime you're feeling
      stressed and need to calm down. Do it anytime you
      think it might help. Don't forget that you're the boss
      of you and that you can do something to calm and
      focus whenever you need to."

Holding Hands involves physical touch, which releases feel-
good hormones in the body and increases focus. Most children
can develop the skill of concentration. Of course, they often
have no problem concentrating on a video game or learning new
features on their smartphones, but nondigital activities such as
focusing on the heartbeat or hands will help them build their attentional skills and increase their mindfulness.

Attention

Concentrate all your thoughts on the work at hand. The sun's rays do not burn until brought to a focus.
ALEXANDER GRAHAM BELL

Paying attention is using your mind's awareness in a focused way. Every healthy adult and child can learn to do this, which means focusing fully on something. We can help sharpen our children's ability to pay attention and observe their thoughts, as well as choose their thoughts, through mindfulness practices. Though mindfulness can be developed through life experiences, the goal here is to help our children hear the whisper of their bodies, minds, and spirits versus "feeling the brick" of life lessons.

My client Chase watched many of his third-grade peers cheat on their weekly spelling quiz, but he didn't feel right about it and decided to take the test honestly. He heard his whisper. His friends, Logan and Cayman, got caught cheating, which landed them in the principal's office. They got the brick of this life lesson, whereas Chase has learned to listen to his own signals.

Mindful Thinking

Mindful Thinking is the process of paying attention to your thoughts and then learning how to choose them. In the first part of the activity, children learn to pay attention to their surroundings and create their thoughts.

USE WHEN

- children get stuck in mental loops
- they make the same careless mistakes repeatedly
- they don't seem to listen to you, or they tune you out

Why the Tools Work

1. Children enjoy the experience of creating their thoughts in a fun way and learning to pay attention to them.

2. Boys and girls are inherent problem solvers, and the second part of the activity, Reframe Game, helps them unstick their thinking about one of their challenges.

3. They are simple but profound activities to help children learn the power of their thoughts and how they are always choosing them.

How to Implement

Mindful Thinking consists of two activities: Anchor Meditation and Reframe Game.

Anchor Meditation

Anchor Meditation goes by many names, but I refer to it this way because it helps children to feel grounded in one place and to state their thoughts about their surroundings. Here are the steps:

1. Select a time and place to be with your child. (In the car on the way to school works well, since he's captive!)

2. Guide your child to start paying attention to his senses. Go through the five senses, and ask each one: What am I _____ right now? Go in this order, if possible: Hearing? Seeing? Touching? Tasting? Smelling?

    Encourage your child to get as specific as possible. For example, if you were in the car, you might say, "I am touching the car, I feel my feet on the floor and my back against the seat. My hands are touching the wheel." You might go through each sense first. For example, you could say, "I smell a cup of coffee," and then ask your child, "What do you smell?" and so on.

If your child is older, you can ask him to name three things instead of just one. For example, you might say, "What three things are you touching right now?" Or "What three things are you seeing right now?" Or "What three things are you hearing right now?"

3. Discuss this activity. Did your child notice things he normally misses?

What You Will Find

Children like to play games, especially ones that seem simple and even silly. The goal here is to raise children's awareness about what's happening around them and let them know that they have the power to observe those things and create their thoughts about them. What they observe is their choice.

Reframe Game

Learning how to reframe a challenge into an opportunity takes practice and mindful thinking. In this activity, I provide guidance for teaching your children how to take a current challenge and see it from other sides. Every situation, even the most challenging ones, can be fodder for your children's positive emotional health.

Follow these steps:

1. Get a few pieces of paper out and place them on the table. Take a piece of paper for yourself, and give one to your child. Draw a box in the middle of the piece of paper like so:

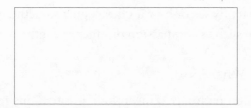

2. On the inside of the box, identify and write down a current challenge you're dealing with — and have your child do the process, too. Some challenging examples for your child might be:

    - My best friend is moving to another state.
    - I'm starting a new school in September and I'm nervous.
    - My classmate is being mean to me.

    Now the problem is inside the box, yet there are four sides to the box. The goal is to see four other sides to this situation, especially the more constructive ones. Let's use the example of "I'm starting a new school in September and I'm nervous" as the challenge. Let's look at it from four new sides.

    - I might meet my new BFF at this school.
    - This school starts later than my old school and I can sleep a bit later.
    - There are lots of after-school activities like volleyball and tennis that I might like.
    - Maybe this school is a good change for me and I might really like it.

3. Discuss with your children. The Reframe Game can guide your children or students to see other sides of their current challenge. Brainstorm how it may be leading them to something good that they can't

currently see or how it's developing something internal, such as compassion or inner strength.

WHAT YOU WILL FIND

Some children naturally want to look at situations from different angles, while others have more difficulty doing so. There's no right or wrong. We all have different learning styles and intelligences, but the ability to see a situation from different perspectives softens challenges and helps children make lemonade out of the lemons in their life. Of course, there are times when a lemon is simply a lemon, but recognizing that is also a part of mindfulness.

Mindful Listening

Paying attention to a particular sound or to someone's speaking is Mindful Listening. Teaching children to place their full awareness on one thing — such as the sound of a bell in the next activity, Mindfulness Bell — can help them cultivate concentration and self-awareness skills.

MINDFULNESS BELL

The goal of this activity is to encourage your children to place their full awareness, even briefly, on the sound of the mindfulness bell. If you have a bell, gong, or singing bowl, you can use that in this activity, or if you're more tech savvy, you can find a mindfulness bell sound on YouTube or on a mindfulness app such as Insight Timer, which is free.

1.   Start by sitting with your child in a calm and comfortable place. Lose all distractions (close the door, and tell everyone you need some quiet time). Introduce the Mindfulness Bell activity by saying you're learning how to become more mindful and you want your child's help.

2. Tell your child that you're going to ring a bell (in person or via technology) that signals both of you to close your eyes. Say, "Listen to the sound of the bell fully. When you no longer hear the bell, open your eyes. Ready?" Ring the bell. (The ring will likely last anywhere between five and thirty-five seconds, depending on the bell). Repeat as often as you like. I like to do five rounds of the Mindfulness Bell early in the day with children so they can calm and get into their mindful listening bodies. There is no right or wrong way to do this. Many people use the mindfulness bell at the beginning and at the end of their meditation sessions with their children, which can be a wonderful way to bookend that type of listening.

3. Discuss this experience.

What You Will Find

Some children are naturally sensitive to sounds, which makes this an activity they might enjoy. Choosing a pleasing sound, perhaps even letting children choose it, is important. The more participation from our children in these activities, the better. Even though some children aren't as inclined to listening to sounds, they can likely benefit the most from this activity because it will help them sharpen their mindful listening skills.

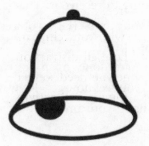

Mindful Giving

Being able to mindfully place your attention on something is a skill, especially as it relates to mindful generosity or giving.

MINDFUL GOODNESS

This activity, Mindful Goodness, is one I often recommend at the end of the day (like at bedtime), because it's calming and can help your child review the day.

1. Be in a quiet and calm place with your child (again, bedtime is perfect). Ask your child to participate in a Mindful Giving exercise with you. You're going to lead your child in an imagining exercise in which you review the day (or recent events) and send people good wishes.

2. Instruct your children like this: "Let's begin. Close your eyes and think of someone who has been nice to you today or recently. Do you have someone in mind?" (If your child has a hard time thinking of someone, help her pick someone, like a teacher or a friend.)

    "Imagine being with that person in your favorite place, and now give her a gift of appreciation for being so good to you. Give her whatever you'd like — flowers, chocolates, a crystal, or something you know she'd love. Imagine the details of giving it to her and her being happy to receive it. This is a gift of good wishes. Take your time." (Give your child a few minutes to imagine this.)

    "When you're done, open your eyes. How did this feel? Did you feel how good it was to give someone something in your mind? To send good mental wishes?"

3.   Discuss with your children and repeat, as desired. "Of course, we can do this again — we can do this for (a) someone you don't like so much and send him or her good wishes, and (b) for people or beings you don't even know. One group of creatures we send good wishes to that's fun is all the animals in the sea or birds in the sky or children on the planet who live in faraway lands and eat different foods. Remember that the good you send out gets returned to you, so even if you don't like someone, you want to send him good wishes, but you don't need to be his friend."

WHAT YOU WILL FIND

Children who expand their concept of giving to include sending good wishes from their minds are learning that they get to choose their thoughts and think mindfully. Helping children realize that generosity can happen in many ways, from sharing a kind word to sending mental good wishes, helps raise their self-awareness and, ultimately, helps them make smarter choices. (Of course, you'll find that most children have a hard time sending good wishes to people they don't like, but when they realize that life is like a boomerang — you get what you send out — they might be more willing to try.)

Centering

At the center of your being you have the answer; you know who you are and you know what you want.

LAO TZU

Centering is the process of coming back to your essence. Your core, your center, is the place within you that is unshaken by outer events, the space that holds who you really are and why you came forth into this time-space reality. Children who can learn to get still and come back to their center, the innermost part of themselves that is clear, calm, and connected, can live the life of their dreams. Your center is a place of emotional balance and strength.

Mindful Meditation

Mindful Meditation teaches children how to calm and center themselves whenever they're able to close their eyes. Centering can happen a number of ways, from taking deep breaths to saying a motto such as "This too shall pass," and boom, you're back in your center, remembering that you're perfect, whole, and complete now.

MINDFUL MEDITATION

Here are the steps and a sample script:

1. "Sit in a comfortable position, whether that's cross-legged on the floor or in a chair. The important thing is that your back is straight, your body is comfortable, and you feel relaxed."

2. "Close your eyes. Of course, you can do this meditation with your eyes open or partially open, but to start let's close your eyes. This helps you shut out any distractions such as funny sounds, smells, sights, and other sensory input."

3. "Focus on your breath. We're going to focus on your breath through a few guided breaths together, which are aimed at helping you center. Come to the place within you that is calm and clear. First take three breaths on your own, nice and slow. Breathe in through the nose, and out through the mouth as if

you're blowing out birthday candles. Do this three times."

4. "Let's breathe together. For the next few breaths, I'll give you some instructions, and it will be easy. First, take a deep breath and breathe in calmness. Think of a calm moment and breathe it in. Hold. Then breathe out frustrations. Let them go. Good. Second breath together, let's breathe in peace and happiness. Imagine all the happy things you love coming into your life. Hold. Then, breathe out unhappy things. Let them go. Well done!"

5. "Third breath together, let's breathe in clarity, the feeling that you know exactly who you are and what you want today. Imagine your perfect day. Breathe it in! Really feel it. Hold. Now, breathe out anything that isn't your perfect day. Let it go. Great job!"

6. "Three more deep breaths, and we're done. Remember, take a breath in your nose, and let it out through your mouth as if you're blowing out birthday candles. Do this three times."

7. "Open your eyes."

8. "Tell me about your experience."

WHAT YOU WILL FIND

Children can do this centering meditation anytime they need to calm and to reconnect with the truth of who they are. There are other centering meditations, especially those involving movement and deep breathing, but the point is to help your children come up with their own activity that helps them center and come back to balance. (Remember to use the breath in any activity as a calming and cooling mechanism, especially for children who run hot.)

Real Kids, Real Stories

A lost coin is found by means of a candle; the deepest truth is found by means of a simple story.

ANTHONY DE MELLO

Children and adults alike learn through stories. We temporarily forget our own lives and get immersed in someone else's story, but in the end, their story is, of course, our story, too. Below I share a few parents' stories of how they've begun teaching mindfulness to their children in creative ways, which hopefully will inspire your own story.

Mindful Touch

Anne, a mom and therapist from Washington, DC, shared with me her story of teaching Mindful Touch. She said, "I hide different items in paper bags and have my children feel them with their eyes closed." One of her bags always has something gooey, which children love, and it brings up many emotions for them.

Keeping their eyes closed, they have to describe and try to identify the object, which also helps build their discomfort tolerance, which is essential for positive emotional health. Often exercises like this seem silly or simple, but they actually have hugely positive results for helping children pay attention and learn to handle unknown situations, even the sticky ones!

Mindful Gratitude

Hana, a mom of four, has a blended family in London. She told me, "It was only when we first started doing this that we found peace in our home, and we believed that anything negative that happened was happening for us to learn from." Hana described to me a mindful exercise of gratitude. Everyone sits on the floor, and they go around the room touching their hearts and sharing a specific thing, person, or situation they're grateful for from that day. Her four-year-old says, "I'm grateful for pancakes," while her stepdaughter says, "I'm grateful for my friend Abby today, who made me smile." Hana happily admits that her family went from a complaining cluster to one that looks for things to appreciate on a daily basis, which certainly nurtures their positive emotional health.

Mindful Car Rides

Chris, father of one, commutes to work daily from New Jersey to New York City. On the way he drops off his son, Samuel, at school, which proves to be a fruitful time for mindfulness. While they're not doing a closed-eye meditation (thankfully), they do set a mindfulness timer using the free app Insight Timer, and they pay attention to things on the ride. Chris told me, "We focus on seeing things of a particular color, and other times we focus on sounds." Along with making the morning commute go by faster, Chris explains that it also creates some fun in the morning and gets his son to start paying attention without staring at a screen. This is the start of mindful seeing.

Mindful Uno

Darsha, a mom from India, says she uses mindfulness daily with her daughter. "I tell her that we create through our thoughts, words, and actions and that she has the power to choose and accept what she wants to create." Her daughter, Bodhi, loves this idea and uses it when playing Uno, the card game. She says, "I choose and accept good cards," and wouldn't you know it — she wins nine out of ten times. What I love about this story is that it encourages Bodhi to realize that she is steering her emotional boat and creating her life — that nobody can do it for her (remember: this is a core idea about emotions from chapter 3).

Mindful Breathing

Matilda, a mom and teacher from Sydney, Australia, has a great way to teach children about Mindful Breathing: "I have them use bubbles. First, they pick up the bubble wand slowly and carefully. They then get to blow one bubble at a time." Of course, this is geared more toward younger children, but I love that she encourages them to go slowly (a sign of mindfulness) and take one deep breath at a time through bubble making. This goes to show that learning mindfulness doesn't have to be dull — it can be fun, too.

Mindful Classrooms

Mindfulness is a powerful tool which supports children in calming themselves, focusing their attention, and interacting effectively with others, all critical skills for functioning well in school and in life.

AMY SALTZMAN

Imagine a classroom full of kindergartners coming back from recess. Instead of being rowdy they listen as they are directed to sit while today's "mindful leader" comes to the front of the room. This leader then leads the whole class in an exercise in which each child says, "I am calm now" and then touches one of their fingers. They do this five times, completing a whole hand and becoming quiet instead. A feeling of calmness descends upon the room. Magic? Not really, but practice and effort? Absolutely. This was a real scenario, which happened in Liz Slade's class in Larchmont, New York, at Chatsworth Elementary School.

Bringing mindfulness into the classroom can help children regulate their emotions and find the calm they need to make smarter choices, choices that have consequences, such as whether to cheat on an exam or speak up about the bullying happening on the playground. Of course, mindfulness cannot solve every problem, but it does help children become more self-aware and often more compassionate, too.

While mindfulness in the classroom is a big win from my perspective, not everyone sees it that same way. One group of parents was so opposed to mindfulness in their Ohio school that they had the program shut down basically because mindfulness — originally — was rooted in Eastern religions. But today's mindfulness in the classroom has nothing to do with religion; it's merely giving children the tools to become self-aware and then make smarter choices.

Complementing mindfulness in the classroom is the formal study of social and emotional learning (SEL). Many schools have to pick either a mindfulness or an SEL program, but honestly one comes before the other. Mindfulness teaches children how to pay attention, which is necessary for SEL ideas, tools, and practices to be effective. An SEL program without an element of mindfulness is like tea without water; it just doesn't work.

While these approaches have similar goals, to help children self-regulate and increase their attentional capabilities, they use different methods for doing so. I perceive SEL to be more intellectual and coming from a cognitive angle (outside in), while I think of mindfulness as more experiential (inside out). Again, these complementary approaches are both helpful, but in an ideal educational world, mindfulness would come first and SEL second.

TAKE NOTE

MINDFULNESS IN THE SCHOOLS

Curricula that teach mindfulness are helping countless children around the globe, but three programs in particular stand out:

Mind Up. The Hawn Foundation (founded by Goldie Hawn) created the Mind Up curriculum for elementary-aged students (K-8). It is informed by neuroscience and teaches how the brain works as well as how to calm and pay attention. I like one of the program's unique features, which is the emphasis on giving children "Brain Breaks" that help them center and calm by closing their eyes and taking a few minutes of silence (www .mindup.org).

Mindful Schools. Mindful Schools offers a curriculum to teach mindfulness in schools, from elementary to high school (K-12). What I like about this curriculum is how accessible it is for teachers to learn remotely, which actually increases the probability that they'll do it and bring it to their classrooms (in public and private schools alike). Mindful Schools also offers a community of educators online to support each other's efforts (www.mindfulschools.org).

Mindfulness in Schools Project (MiSP). A UK-based organization, MiSP aims to bring mindfulness to UK students to foster their well-being. They host conferences and are the leading provider of mindfulness curricula in the UK (for seven- to eighteen-year-olds) (www.mindfulnessinschools.org).

Mindfulness and Character

Human greatness does not lie in wealth or power, but in character and goodness.

ANNE FRANK

Mindfulness teaches us to pay attention without wanting to run to or from something. It is simply observing and accepting what is. With time, any adult or child who practices mindfulness can become more aware of his or her thoughts, feelings, and actions. Such awareness leads most people to want to become better, which promotes the formation of a more honest, kind, and compassionate character.

Said differently, mindfulness doesn't make you a better person, but it does help you become aware of who you are and where your choices are leading you. When we see ourselves without filters, most of us want to make changes — such as becoming more generous or forgiving — which is healthy. These are qualities of *character*, which Oxford Living Dictionaries defines as "the mental and moral qualities distinctive to an individual."

Scholars and scientists have shown that mindfulness cultivates the inner quality of compassion in most children. This type of kindness naturally rises up when you realize that everyone has pain and that everyone wants to be free of it. Empathy is when you feel what someone else is feeling. It is not as advanced as compassion, but it's a good starting point to feel what someone else is feeling. Compassion goes a step further by not only seeing Jackson on the playground hit Billy but wanting Jackson to stop. You feel what someone is feeling, and then you want him to be free of pain — this is compassion, and it's a contributor to positive emotional health.

Mindfulness helps children become more self-aware and, as a result, most realize that it's in their best interest to make choices that are good for them and good for others. This is how character is built. Having an honest and kind character also contributes mightily to your child's positive emotional health (most children don't stay awake wondering, *Was I too honest?* But children do lie awake thinking, *Maybe I shouldn't have cheated on that exam*).

Cultivating Character

As we know, raising emotionally healthy children begins with helping them identify their emotions and then learning how to constructively express them. This is step one. This process becomes even more important when children go to school and experience conflict (bullies, failed exams, feeling left out, frenemies). But on a parallel path we also need to help a child become a good person — the type of person who opens the door for others and shares his lunch if his friend forgot hers.

Becoming this good person is based on cultivating certain inner qualities or characteristics, which can be helped along by mindfulness. The top six that positively impact a child's emotional health are:

GRATITUDE	A thought of appreciation and a feeling of thankfulness, which help children realize how good things already are.
COMPASSION	When a child not only feels what someone else is feeling (empathy) but wants their pain to stop. For example, Billy doesn't just notice Mark struggling with his backpack and crutches; Billy offers to carry Mark's backpack.
GENEROSITY	A child who learns to give because it feels good and helps others is generous. She's not doing it to get something back but simply because it is kind and good.

HONESTY	To speak and act truthfully. An honest child is learning that what goes around comes around, and since he doesn't want anyone lying to him, he'll need to be honest, too.
FORGIVENESS	A child who forgives is learning to let go of negative emotions about a wrongdoing that will only make her miserable. For example, Ella's sister cracked her iPad case, but Ella forgave her and said, "Accidents happen."
LOVE	A loving child is learning how to fully love herself and extend that kindness to others. That doesn't mean she's friends with everyone, but she can let others earn her affections.

These qualities nurture positive emotional health, helping to bring a child back to balance. Andy, at age eight, gets angry easily and stomps his feet repeatedly at home. But when his mom, Tricia, says, "I need you to tell me five thankful things, and then we can talk," Andy names five things, from his new pet fish, Peyton, to his neighbor, Jackson. And guess what? His anger softens and he's more amenable to listening and connecting.

The raising of emotionally healthy children is done from the outside in, through teaching ideas and tools (SEL), and also from the inside out, through mindfulness and character building, so that children can move with gusto toward their healthiest and happiest lives. Other important factors that impact a child's growing sense of well-being are:

- sense of humor
- friendships
- body care (eating, sleeping, getting exercise)
- after-school activities

A child's ability to make not only healthy friendships but also smart choices is facilitated by mindfulness and character development. What I see as one of the most challenging parts of humanity is a lack of honesty. We have all told white lies, but if we can help children learn that what they send out comes back to them — think the law of cause and effect, the golden rule, karma — they can begin to make choices that are more truthful and in their best interest.

Olivia, age eleven, lied to her best friend, Ava. Ava was trying out for her class's second-grade talent contest, and Olivia was to be in charge of the music while Ava danced. In the middle of Ava's tap-dancing routine, the music went silent and Olivia looked surprised. But the truth of the matter was that Olivia was jealous, pulled the plug on the music intentionally, and wanted Ava to mess up. After I coached Olivia, she apologized to Ava and amazingly enough, Ava forgave her.

Learning how to repair relationships (especially in middle school) is essential to developing positive emotional health and making (as well as keeping) healthy friendships. The lesson Olivia learned is that honesty really is the best policy, and I hope she doesn't need to learn it again.

Mindful Technology

The opportunities are amazing for the touch-screen generation.

DEVORAH HEITNER

Learning how to use technology, without being used by it, is an essential skill we need to teach our children. Of course, teaching this requires that we model healthy screen-time and digital-device use, too. I heard one mom say, "My daughter asked if stoplights were created so we can check our email," and she laughed. Just because we can be connected doesn't necessarily mean it's the healthiest thing for us — or for our children to see.

But technology can also be a tool of mindfulness. Of course, as a digital immigrant (not born with an iPad), I find being around digital natives to be hilarious. They seem to come hardwired for the use of devices, and they know — just know — how computers work. When I got my new iPhone, the person at the Apple store asked if I'd like to attend a Genius Bar session about how to use it, and I laughed because I thought, *Who is it taught by? An eight-year-old? They're the ones who really know the tips and tricks.*

While many children may know how technology works, that doesn't mean they use it mindfully — and most need to be mentored in how to do this. Devorah Heitner, author of *Screenwise*, suggests that it's parents and teachers who can help children build their healthy habits around screens, and I couldn't agree more. And since technology isn't going away and can be used for the good, I've decided to highlight some of the mindfulness-related tech that has been found to be helpful to children (and their parents!).

Apps

- *Headspace* (www.headspace.com/kids) helps children meditate, calm, sleep, focus, be kind, and wake up. I have used this with children, and they love it.
- *Stop, Breathe & Think* (www.stopbreathethink.com /kids) helps children focus, calm, and sleep (for children five to ten years old).
- *Smiling Mind* (www.smilingmind.com.au) provides free tools, such as the body scan, to help your children become mindful and relaxed.

- *Calm* (www.calm.com) helps adults and children relax and sleep better. There are many free guided meditations.

Parental Wi-Fi Controls

While these are not necessarily mindfulness-based technologies, they can help us become more mindful about how much time we as adults spend on our screens and allow our children to do the same. I'm a big fan of role-modeling healthy technology use, making agreements, and having rules for the whole family, and these tools can help.

- *Circle* (www.meetcircle.com) by Disney helps parents turn on and off their children's devices from afar, as well as filter content, and set a time for when Wi-Fi goes on and off in the house.
- *Koalasafe* (www.koalasafe.com) is another internet control device, which helps parents block sites, monitor usage, and schedule Wi-Fi time limits.

TAKE NOTE

SOME LOW-TECH TOOLS

Nurturing mindfulness in your children can be done in a low-tech way, too. Here are some low-tech tools:

- **Mindfulness Matters** (www.playtherapysupply.com) is a card deck I've used with older children; it's recommended for children nine to eighteen years old. Every card has a question that can be a mindful conversation starter.
- **Mad Dragon** (www.childtherapytoys.com) is an anger-control card game for children six to twelve years old. It

comes highly recommended by school counselors who help children cultivate self-awareness, especially around anger.

- **Self-Control Thumball** (www.playtherapysupply.com) is a small ball covered with prompts about self-control, which is a skill of emotional health facilitated by mindfulness.

Of course, there are books on mindfulness and other tools that can help you foster your child's growing sense of self-awareness, but let's not forget — anything your child does with her full focus can help her concentrate and become more mindful, even washing your car!

Top Ten Mindfulness Tips

When teaching mindfulness to your children (or classroom) it's important to go slowly and take one step at a time. This doesn't need to be a New Year's resolution that you'll throw out by February but something easy that you'll follow through on. So to help you put mindfulness into practice, below I provide my top ten tips for getting started:

1. *Start slow.* Learn about mindfulness, and carefully select the type of mindfulness practice you'd like to begin with your children. Some examples may be breathing, walking, mindful moving, listening, and seeing.

2. *Pick one thing.* If we pick one thing and stick to it, we'll make progress. My one thing is meditation because it calms, centers, and helps me connect to guidance. But my one thing needn't be yours. You can use mindful breathing or calming audios to help your child prepare for bedtime, for example.

3. *Use technology to your benefit.* Using mindfulness apps or audios can help our children calm and pay better attention. I personally use a mindfulness app, which records my daily meditation and connects me to a community of folks who are meditating at the same time.

4. *Recognize that you can always begin again.* Wiping the slate clean and beginning again is one of the philosophies of mindfulness. There is no need to carry the past or to fear the future with mindfulness, which is always happening in the present. Often children need do-overs, which mindfulness encourages and teaches us to embrace. Because honestly, we can always begin again, no matter what.

5. *Create a nightly mindfulness practice that helps you and your child.* It may be something simple like reading *Goodnight Moon* and saying goodnight and thank you to every person you saw that day. Or perhaps it's Tool 5 (page 82), in which you place your hand on your heart and connect with your breathing to relax. Or maybe every evening you sit with your child and list your Five Joys from the day, which I love. This is particularly helpful because it trains your child's mind to begin looking for the good things life has to offer.

6. *Connect with mindful schools and/or communities.* Connect with communities where mindfulness is valued, taught, and lived. One place like that in my Santa Barbara community is Yoga Soup, which offers mindfulness-based yoga for children and their parents.

7. *Use mindfulness daily.* Sometimes as parents and teachers we think we have to "fix it" when a child is

angry. We have him take deep breaths, or we tell him to listen to his calming audios when he can't sleep. Those aren't bad ideas, but I want to encourage you to use mindfulness practices when your child feels good, not just at challenging times or on hard days. It's the regular habit that makes it really work and helps children remember to take deep breaths when they need them.

8. *Make mindful friends.* Do your best to help your son or daughter make friends who are mindful, considerate, and thoughtful. If possible, take your child to activities where other mindful children may be — for example, karate or art class. The possibilities are endless, but certainly having a peer who makes a positive impact on your child is a good thing.

9. *Realize that mindfulness takes time, and be in it for the long haul.* No quick fixes here, or as they say, no McMindfulness. Mindfulness is about slowing down, not doing things quickly. Early in my life a teacher told me, "Slow down to get where you want to go faster," and that made an impression on me. After all, the tortoise won the race, not the hare.

10. *Get a mindfulness mentor.* Mentors are people who are farther along the path of mindfulness than you are. Your mentor doesn't even need to be someone you know — it could be His Holiness the Dalai Lama, and maybe you watch his videos, read his books, or learn from his teachings. It doesn't need to be a spiritual teacher, either, but someone like Jon Kabat-Zinn, who wrote *Full Catastrophe Living* and *Wherever You Go, There You Are.*

Mindfulness is a wonderful way of living in this world, but I don't want to underestimate the power of "mindlessness" either. Our bodily functions (like breathing) happen automatically without any thought. The ability to be mindless, or to empty our minds, and just relax to restore ourselves has its role, too. Learning how to go from mindless to mindful is what we want to teach our children, which is healthy — it's a balance.

Scratching the Surface

Being a parent is one of the greatest mindfulness practices of all.

JON KABAT-ZINN

Mindfulness is a sophisticated subject, which you can study throughout your whole life as you continue to deepen your ability to be mindful. Within these pages, I've shared an introduction to mindfulness with a special focus on helping our children learn how to pay attention in this certain way and without judgment. Below I share some other qualities of mindfulness, which you can explore over time, if you're so inclined:

- self-compassion
- discipline (stick-with-it-ness)
- playfulness
- lightness of touch

Lightness of touch, a term used by Kabat-Zinn, can be understood as being demonstrated by a person who is gentle with himself, others, and the world. He doesn't come into a room screaming and leave slamming the door but recognizes that power resides in the strength of being calm and connected. He's emotionally balanced, which means he's not at the extremes of either anger or sadness but content in the middle.

Helping children find the middle, or their center, is precisely what mindfulness practices can do. Siya, age eight, hates to go to bed. Her mom decided to create a "mindful moment" before bedtime, so they sit facing each other and they hit a chime in her bedroom. Then they take a few deep breaths and share what they're grateful for that day. Since Siya loves to review her day, she has started to look forward to this bedtime ritual and even sleeps better now. She has found a way to center.

Using mindfulness as a tool to help your child calm, come back to center, and ultimately, make smarter choices is enlightened parenting. It's bringing light to this sometimes dark and challenging world for your children. It's also introducing them to a way of being that they can learn about throughout their lives.

Up Next

I pride myself on being practical, so the next chapter, "The Toolbox," shares many common childhood emotions and tools to help your child come back to center — to discover her emotional balance. Becoming emotionally healthy and positive isn't always easy in this stressful world, but with tools, time, and practice, it is certainly possible for nearly everyone.

Part Three

HABITS

Chapter Six

THE TOOLBOX

You're only as strong as the tools in your toolbox.
MICHAEL BASTIAN

Yesterday my neighbor was assembling his daughter's "big-girl bed" from Santa Claus. I know because in the midst of this project, he knocked on my door looking for a tool, which I loaned him. Emotions work the same way. Without the correct tools, a happier and more productive life cannot be constructed. Some of the tools of positive emotional health are mindfulness, breathing, and centering, which, as we've seen, can take many forms.

Nora, age six, is my neighbor's eldest daughter. She gets very scared going into dark places in her home. I taught her to say, "I am brave, I am safe, and I am guided" to help her diminish her fear if she needed to go into a dark room and turn on the light. Her mindful self-talk has really boosted her confidence and helped her navigate scary situations. Of course, this is just one tool in her toolbox.

Helping children recognize how emotions work and what tools to use in different scenarios empowers them. They can face their fears, just as Nora learned to handle her discomfort with the dark and just as my client Atticus, who tends to worry, whether boarding a train or taking a big test, has learned ways to cope. Of course, the good news is that the tools that work for our children usually work for us, too.

A few weeks ago, I was crossing an epic bridge on Route 154 in California with straight drops into the Los Padres National Forest on both sides, which scared me. I used the same "I am safe" mantra as I drove over it, which helped reduce my discomfort. When our children see us use a tool it helps them, too. They realize we're in it together and that everyone has big feelings they're learning to express constructively.

In this chapter, we continue our discussion of how to stop, calm, and make smarter choices with awareness. Some of the tools below we've discussed already, while others are new. All are alphabetized by emotion. My goal is for this chapter to be an easy-to-use resource that allows you to look up an emotion (for example, anger, sadness, and worry) and be given a tool to help immediately. Of course, every child is different, but this section provides a starting point for on-the-spot nurturing of positive emotional health.

Cracking the Code

In the upcoming toolbox I use a system of codes to indicate whether the emotion is one to increase (+), since it is helpful for your child's positive emotional health, or whether it's one that is challenging (-), which needs to be reduced (or more accurately, transformed) through constructive self-expression. Of course, every emotion needs constructive expression, but some, like gratitude and enthusiasm, are affirmative by their very nature.

You may notice that I'm steering away from labeling emotions as either good or bad (negative), since every emotion can be used for good; it's how we express it that matters. Along with codes I also provide:

- a definition
- tools
- a list of similar emotions

One of the reasons I define each emotion, although the definitions may look simplistic, is that I have found over the years that when I say "empathy," for example, people may think a certain thing, which may not be what I mean. I provide a short commentary as well.

TAKE NOTE

A STARTING POINT

Children might need to learn a smorgasbord of tools before they find the one that works for them, such as Tool 5 (Hand on Heart) or Tool 4 (Bubble Breathing). Or they might learn the tools in this book and then create their own version. For example, when I taught Missy, a ten-year-old client, Bubble Breathing, she came up with Flower Petal Breathing, in which she smelled a flower (in her imagination) and then blew out air onto the petals, which made her feel better. Of course, children are infinitely creative, which is one of the reasons I adore them. So please use the tools in this book as a starting point for building your child's emotional toolbox.

Anger (-)

The feeling of intense frustration and discontent. The emotionally healthy child needs to find constructive outlets for his or her anger. As we've discussed, this is a fast-moving emotion, and many children respond quickly to the feeling of anger. Some of the solutions to anger management include slowing down, stopping, and calming before reacting negatively. Common scenarios in which many children get angry are: being told to turn off their digital device and being told to complete their homework.

Since anger is such a fast-moving emotion, one of the keys to success is having your child slow down and stop before making not-so-smart choices. (Remember: *We must get them physically calm before they can think calmer thoughts.*)

Tools

- *Awareness:* Tool 1 (Volcano), Tool 2 (Anger Buttons), Tool 3 (Anger Name)
- *Breathing:* Tool 4 (Bubble Breathing), Mindful Breathing (Five for Five) on page 117, Finger Tracing Breath (below) and Two Languages (below)
- *Self-Talk:* Sayings such as "This too shall pass" can help children remember that anger comes and goes. They don't have to react to it but can let it pass by like clouds in the sky.
- *Outlets:* This can be something physical like hitting a punching bag or something creative like coloring.

Similar Emotions

Madness, rage, frustration, hostility, annoyance

Scenario

Charles, father of three children, told me how he helps his five-year-old son, Billy, calm after getting angry. Billy looks at one hand and uses his other hand to trace his hand while taking a deep breath at each finger. After two or three rounds, he feels calmer and starts to let the anger go (tool: Finger Tracing Breath).

Sophia, a single mom, shared with me how she helps her daughter get calm by asking her to count to ten first in English and then in Spanish (*uno, dos, tres, cuatro*) (tool: Two Languages). Each of these scenarios involves getting the right and left brain working together, thus slowing down the big emotions and bringing logic online sooner.

Bravery (+)

The feeling of courage. The emotionally healthy child is learning how to muster his or her sense of bravery to face big emotions and learn how to master them. Challenging emotions come with a level of discomfort, which children need to learn to tolerate and embrace with the awareness that they're bigger than any emotion, even the uncomfortable ones. Cultivating courage can happen in many different ways, but tools and practice help enormously.

Tools

- *Breathing:* Tool 4 (Bubble Breathing) and Nose Breath (below)
- *Self-Talk (affirmations):* Ask your child to use "I am" statements such as "I am brave" and "I am safe" to bolster her courage, especially when she's faced with a new situation.
- *Visualization:* Lead children in seeing themselves as brave and as having "superhero" power from the inside out. (See my prior book, *Growing Happy Kids.*)

Similar Emotions

Courage, confidence, grit, perseverance, inner strength

Scenario

Amy, mother of three children, says helping them "feel and be brave" is an everyday occurrence. Her ten-year-old, Ben, just started at a new school, and together they used nostril breathing to calm him each day before school. They take a deep breath through the nose, hold it for three seconds, and let it out through the mouth (tool: Nose Breathing). Amy said, "It takes about three to five rounds for Ben to calm, but he does!"

After mindful breathing, Amy continues to help bolster Ben's sense of courage and his ability to make new friends. They do "I am" statements such as "I am brave, I am courageous, I am making new friends, and I am feeling good." Ben reluctantly plays along, but after a few "I am" statements he stands taller and begins to have fun, laughing and making up his own sayings. Amy and Ben have also visualized Ben making new friends.

Calm (+)

The feeling of serenity or peace. The emotionally healthy child is learning how to bring him- or herself back to calm after feeling challenged. Deep within the center of every person is a place of peace and calm that cannot be touched by this world, and learning how to connect to this space is calming. You needn't be religious to close your eyes and feel the calmness that resides within.

Tools

- *Breathing:* (Five for Five) on page 117 and Gorilla Breath and Child's Pose (below)

- *Calming:* Tool 4 (Bubble Breathing) and Tool 5 (Hand on Heart)
- *Outlets (creative or physical):* Tool 11 (Color It Out)

Similar Emotions

Quiet, stillness, connection, serenity, peace

Scenario

Eddie, a yoga teacher, told me how he helps children use both parts of their brains in calming. He gave me two new mindful movements, which help children get their energy out and create calmness:

> *Gorilla Breath:* Imagine you're a gorilla walking around taking deep breaths, and even pounding your chest because you're angry. Sway to each side and let your angry energy out. Walk around like a gorilla and really feel the emotions leaving you. Even make noises like an angry gorilla, and let those big feelings go.
>
> *Child's Pose:* A traditional yoga posture that is very effective in helping a child or an adult calm. Put your knees and forehead on the ground while placing your arms palm up behind you. Eyes are typically closed, and breathing slows and calms down. This helps a child come back to the present moment, where all his or her power is.

Compassion (+)

The feeling of feeling someone's pain and wanting him to be free of it. The emotionally healthy child not only empathizes (feels someone else's pain) but wants others not to suffer. For example, Billy saw his best friend struggling with his knapsack and crutches, so instead of watching him struggle he carried his friend's knapsack. Another way compassion is explained is "kindness in action"; it has not only a thinking and feeling aspect but often an action-oriented one as well.

Children who have had challenges, whether it's a physical illness or a loss, often have learned to transform their pain into compassion. Self-compassion is important, too.

Tools

- *Mindfulness:* Especially Mindful Seeing on page 119 and Mindful Goodness on page 130
- *Helping others:* For example, volunteering with parents or doing something nice for someone in your community who can use assistance, like an elderly neighbor
- *Wisdom teachings:* Stories across cultures and countries on compassion

Similar Emotions

Empathy, kindness, forgiveness, love, generosity

Scenario

Keisha, a mom from London, explained to me, "I'm constantly helping my son, Clayton, become more compassionate." He's four years old, and just yesterday she helped him understand that everyone has feelings, especially animals. Apparently, he'd pull their dog's tail and also poke worms in the park with sticks. But after learning about compassion and the "boomerang effect" — what you give out gets returned to you — he stopped annoying the animals and began being nicer to them.

But Keisha wanted Clayton to be kind and compassionate to people, too. She found a local soup kitchen, which has a family volunteering night to help children help others and, ultimately, become more kind. Keisha says, "This experience has been amazing."

Confidence (+)

The feeling of certainty and assuredness. The emotionally healthy child is learning how to develop a healthy sense of confidence. Too much confidence can become arrogance, and too little becomes doubt or uncertainty about one's skills or ability to persevere. (See my earlier book *Growing Happy Kids* about how to create inner confidence.)

Tools

- *Self-Talk:* The thoughts you say to yourself in the privacy of your mind, especially mottos
- *Visualization:* Learning to see oneself as capable takes practice. Lead your child to see him- or herself as successful already. (One of my teachers would say, "If you can see it, you can be it!")
- *Wisdom teachings:* For example, Ernest Holmes, a wise teacher said, "Today I am filled with confidence and a sense of security because I am actively aware of the presence of Spirit within me."

Similar Emotions

Assuredness, certainty, faith in self

Scenario

Lisa, age eleven, exudes confidence, despite having dwarfism and being only three feet tall. When she was asked to speak on her first day of school, Lisa got up in front of the whole school assembly, and said, "I am a little person. I have big feelings like everyone here and have interests. At home, I have a pony, a llama, and a pig in the farm behind my house. Let's talk about animals. Please treat me like everyone else, because I am just like you."

Standing there in the assembly, I was amazed at her confidence and her ability to stand tall in a room full of strangers. When I got a chance to meet Lisa, I asked her: "How are you so confident in front of people?" She said, "My parents teach me to speak up and take control of my life. They tell me I can do anything and that being little is a superpower." I smiled from ear to ear because her parents had helped her think confident thoughts and speak them to herself — and now she feels them, too.

Lisa also told me that she "imagines everything going well" before speaking and standing up for herself. The power of visualization can be game-changing for confidence.

Enthusiasm (+)

The feeling of eager interest. The emotionally healthy child is learning to master his or her emotions while pursuing interests with enthusiasm. Enthusiasm is a helpful emotion because it is closely aligned with joy, happiness, learning, and growth. The child who can discover her interests early on can build her skills and contribute her gifts to the world sooner rather than later.

Tools

- *Mindful language:* Be careful to use language that supports your child's growing interests, and to encourage them, even with interests that don't become lifelong pursuits.

- *Enthusiasm list:* Help your child make a list of things she feels interested in. Be open to interests she may never have expressed before, such as cooking, horseback riding, and robotics. The point is to help children find things to feel enthusiastic about and to encourage them to explore them (formally or informally).
- *Connection:* Make sure your child's friendships and community are encouraging.

Similar Emotions

Interest, passion, motivation, excitement, eagerness

Scenario

Parker, a ten-year-old, came to me because she struggles with her emotions. She has what I would consider an "artistic temperament," which means she's highly sensitive and responds quickly to her feelings. Her parents, Angela and Jack, want to help her learn how to manage her emotions better, which she certainly can do.

Despite her roller-coaster feelings, Parker has great talents, especially in the world of acting, having already been in many commercials and being the lead actress for a local theater company. I recognized this as a great outlet for her enormous and fast-moving energy.

Along with learning some tools to calm (breathing, movement), and applying her Smart Choices Checklist when feeling challenged, Parker poured her energy into being the new lead actress for the upcoming play, *Annie*. Her parents encouraged her, and Parker's enthusiasm was palpable when she made new friends and pursued her interest in an enjoyable way.

Forgiveness (+)

The feeling of releasing grudges or resentments. The emotionally healthy child doesn't only learn to say, "I'm sorry" and be forgiven but learns how to forgive others. Forgiveness, as we know, is a complex subject, but helping children learn to pardon others is necessary for their own mental and emotional health. This doesn't mean condoning what others have done but letting go of grudges so that children can focus on being their emotionally healthiest selves.

Self-forgiveness is probably one of the hardest things for children and adults to do, but it is also necessary on the path to becoming emotionally healthier and happier.

Tools

- *Learn from others:* See my *Psychology Today* article, "Forgiveness" www.psychologytoday.com/us/blog/creative-development/201009/forgiveness.
- *Forgiveness exercises:* Journaling (below) and another bedtime tool, asking, "Was there anyone you held outside of your heart today?" And if the answer is yes, work to forgive that person nightly.

Similar Emotions

Pardon, grace, mercy, absolution

Scenario

Charlie, age eleven, broke his mom's favorite vase. Even though she had told him multiple times not to run around the dining room, he did so anyway and knocked into the cabinet, sending the vase into the air and then into a million pieces. Thankfully, no one was hurt, and Charlie immediately apologized to his mom and said he'd save up to buy her a new one (which wasn't possible but was a nice thought).

Jessica, Charlie's mom, said, "I know this was an accident and that you're sorry, but I'm going to need some time to forgive you." Of course, she's doing the best she can to forgive her son. Where I jumped in was to help Charlie, my client, forgive himself. I helped Charlie understand that mistakes happen and that he needs to be more careful, but also that he must forgive himself to be healthy and happier. To get the ball rolling on self-forgiveness, Charlie promised to write in his electronic journal, "I forgive myself for _____" and then to explore his thoughts on forgiving himself.

Frustration (-)

The feeling of annoyance. The emotionally healthy child is learning how to tolerate discomfort and minor annoyances while constructively expressing them. As you likely know, frustration is a precursor to anger. The goal isn't to remove frustration or annoyances but simply to help your son or daughter learn how to cope with them instead of making not-so-smart choices.

Tools

- *Mindful moment:* Role-model a "sacred pause" in which you close your eyes and take deep breaths when frustrated so you can show your child how to let frustration go.
- *Calming exercises:* Tool 4 (Bubble Breathing) and Tool 5 (Hand on Heart)
- *Outlets:* Tool 11 (Color It Out) or other creative or

physical endeavors like hitting a punching bag or jumping on a trampoline.

Similar Emotions

Annoyance, irritation, disappointment, anger

Scenario

Alex, age ten, gets frustrated regularly in his math class. He got in trouble for throwing pencils, erasers, and his notebook when he struggled with assignments. Of course this isn't acceptable third-grade behavior.

Connecting with Alex, I helped him learn to spot his frustration in his body when it was small, and then stop before throwing things. We did a body scan (Tool 8) for where he feels frustration in his body and identified his warning signs. He said, "I start making fists and my heart beats faster." Helping your child spot frustration when it's small is essential to helping him or her make better choices.

I also shared experiences from my own life when I get frustrated so we could connect and attune over the experience. It's just part of living on this planet. We then did the Smart Choices Checklist (Tool 7) to help Alex identify what he can do when he's feeling frustrated that will produce better results than throwing things, especially in the classroom!

Generosity (+)

The feeling of giving. The emotionally healthy child is learning how to be generous with his or her thoughts, words, and actions. Science reveals that generosity is linked to happiness and that people who give more are typically more content. This isn't rocket science, but we can help children be generous, whether it's giving a child in need some toys or sharing a smile with someone who needs one.

Tools

- *Gratitude exercises* (see "Gratitude")
- *Mindful giving:* Giving your time, attention, or money to help others, as in Mindful Goodness, on page 130
- *Wisdom teachings:* For example, Winston Churchill said, "We make a living by what we get, but we make a life by what we give."

Similar Emotions

Giving, kindness, sharing, altruism, compassion

Scenario

Addison, age seven, lived in a town near a mudslide that displaced thousands of children her age. She felt strongly that her second-grade classroom needed to do something, and she met with her teacher, Mrs. Nancy. At age seven, Addy had a ton of ideas about ways to help, from a bake sale to a movie night (to get children distracted) to a clothes drive. They agreed on a clothes drive, which collected lightly used or new clothes to help 250 children in grades K-5 who were displaced and without their regular clothes.

This clothing drive was such a success that Principal Dan publicly recognized Addison at the school assembly and gave her the Generosity Award for outstanding citizenship and charity. She got a standing ovation and told me, "I loved helping other kids. I can't imagine how hard it is."

Gratitude (+)

The feeling of appreciation. The emotionally healthy child is learning to appreciate whatever shows up in life. Gratitude is a slow-moving emotion, which requires careful tending to increase the feeling of thankfulness and appreciation. Think of gratitude as a muscle. If a young bodybuilder wants to be a world champion, he needs to work out his muscles, and the same is true for gratitude.

Tools

- *Gratitude exercises:* Writing in a gratitude journal (hard copy or electronic) and spending time before dinner going around the table, each stating something to be grateful for, for example
- *Helping others* (less fortunate)
- *Gratitude app:* Three Good Things is a gratitude app that has been scientifically proven to pave positive pathways in the brain by *daily* helping your child identify three good things that happened that day. (Three Good Things: A Happiness Journal is free on iTunes.com.)

Similar Emotions

Thankfulness, appreciation, happiness

Scenario

Grace, age ten, lives in Australia, and I work with her via Skype. Her mom, Alice, contacted me because Grace was crying in the classroom and her school had run out of solutions. After I spent some time with Grace, it became clear that she was a highly emotional child with great gifts but that she needed to learn how to slow down, direct her feelings, and see how good things really are.

Her first step was doing deep breaths and learning how to calm herself. She was in the habit of feeling something (a little discomfort) and reacting quickly, whether this was in the form of tears, saying not-so-nice things, or leaving the classroom. Along with deep breaths, we did the Smart Choices Checklist (Tool 7) so she could make better choices, which did help.

But what I think changed everything for Grace was starting a gratitude journal, which helped her focus on the good things happening. She wasn't in the habit of looking for the positive things every day, so writing about the things she was thankful for changed her mood and how she responds to challenges.

Guilt (-)

The feeling of having done something wrong. The emotionally healthy child is learning how to make mistakes, apologize, and not carry the heavy emotion of guilt. Annie broke her father's glasses and felt guilty about it. She then apologized, took responsibility, and even though she got a consequence, the heavy feeling of guilt left her. This is healthy.

However, using guilt as a motivator for children to do something is emotionally unhealthy and sets up a child for emotional imbalances.

Tools

- *Wisdom teachings:* For example, Wayne Dyer said, "Releasing guilt is like removing a huge weight from your shoulders. Guilt is released through the empowering thought of love and respect for yourself."

- *Mentoring:* Talking to someone and getting wise advice (therapy, mentoring, reading)
- *Outlets:* (physical or creative)

Similar Emotions

Shame, disgrace, feeling of wrongdoing

Scenario

Margarita, age eleven, is the child of divorced parents. She spends a week with her mom and then a week with her dad, per their custody agreement. Margarita said, "I feel so guilty having fun with Dad when Mom's not here." She continued by saying how her dad has a lot of money, and they fly on private planes around the world, while her mom is working 24-7 at the hospital. Helping Margarita realize that both her parents love her and that she has nothing to feel guilty (or wrong) about when she's with one parent helped reduce her guilt.

Guilt is a tricky emotion to help children with because often it's a result of misperceptions on their part or feeling bad for something they've done. When your child says, "I feel bad about _____," this is a sign that she may be carrying guilt, which needs to be released. Of course, regret and remorse are healthy reactions if a mistake has genuinely been made, but guilt is unhealthy.

Happiness (+)

The feeling of joy. The emotionally healthy child is learning what makes him happy, whether it's an ice-cream cone (temporary happiness) or making friendships that bring him contentment (lasting happiness). He's learning to go within to create a deeper type of happiness and is moving forward on the path of positive emotional health. (See my prior book *Growing Happy Kids* for more on this.)

Tools

- *Outlets:* Exercising and pursuing interests for self-expression
- *Connection:* Strong friendships and community to foster happiness (lasting, not fleeting)
- *Helping others* (see "Compassion")
- *Gratitude* (see "Gratitude")
- *Humor:* Having a child-aged joke ready such as "What is a bear without teeth? A gummy bear!"

Similar Emotions

Joy, optimism, hope, gratitude, compassion, kindness, generosity, enjoyment

Scenario

Eden, age eight, was unhappy about her new baby brother. She told me, "He's taking up my parents' time, and they're ignoring me." Of course, change can be challenging, especially adjusting to a new baby brother when beforehand Eden had been an only child. I helped Eden focus on the positive side of this gift, including listing many of Samuel's good qualities, which today consisted of being cute and smiling.

Eden also wasn't getting enough exercise, time with her friends, and opportunities to help others. When we added these to the mix, especially enrolling her in a weekly hip-hop dance class, an after-school sewing class with her best friend, and quarterly volunteering opportunities with her temple, her happiness level bumped up a notch.

Hate (-)

The feeling of extreme dislike. The emotionally healthy child is learning not to grow the emotion of hate, which immediately takes him or her off-balance. Of course, it is one thing to hate carrots or your parents' music, but it's another to hate a person. The opposite of hate isn't love but tolerance. Raising our children to respect differences and to resolve conflicts amicably while seeking common ground is part of nurturing positive emotional health.

Tools

- *Mentoring:* Emotional coaching is needed to dissolve hate and remove ignorance.
- *Conflict resolution:* Many US schools have implemented a "restorative justice" approach to help children become cooperative and tolerant of others.
- *Wisdom teachings:* For example, Martin Luther King Jr. said, "I've decided to stick with love. Hate is too great a burden to bear."

Similar Emotions

Dislike, disgust, disapproval, animosity, resentment, loathing

Scenario

Karen, the mother of three girls, was struggling with her tween, Angie. When Angie got angry she would say, "I hate you, Mom." Not only were these words hurtful for Karen, but she didn't know how to help her daughter control her emotions, settle down her anger, and learn to get along in a positive, cooperative way.

Meeting with Karen and Angie, I helped them establish some ground rules of what they could say to each other and what was off-limits, such as "I hate you." If either of them used the off-limits words, they were required to put $5 into the vacation fund jar

— and if Angie continued on the same track, she'd be taking the whole family to Disneyland soon. But with some focus on skill building, Angie and her mom began improving their communication and relationship.

Specifically, we began doing mindfulness exercises to slow Angie down and help her make better choices when she was frustrated and feeling intense dislike. Karen and Angie also began taking yoga classes together, which helped them bond and reduced outbursts for both of them!

Hope (+)

The feeling that something positive is going to happen. The emotionally healthy child has difficult days but works at never losing hope. Hope is essential for positive emotional health. Without hope a person becomes sad and listless, and life feels not worth living. Many would consider this kind of extreme sadness clinical depression.

Hope comes from understanding the preciousness of life and believing that everything can change in a positive direction, especially if we focus there. Hope places the locus of control within a child, not outside him or her.

Tools

- *Three good things:* Help your child identify three good things that have happened each day, which can help him or her see the good things occurring now. Focusing on the positive can help build hope that things will get better.
- *Mentoring:* Sharing stories of hope, inspiration, and truth from your life or others
- *Optimism exercises:* Tool 6, Wheel of Feel, can be used to move toward feeling more hopeful.

Similar Emotions

Faith, optimism, positive expectation

Scenario

Jessie is fourteen and her dad, Nathan, is battling cancer. Nathan has put on a good face and keeps telling his family, "Keep the faith, I'm going to beat this." Jessie is struggling with staying positive, which she doesn't need to do all the time, but if she can hold some hope that things can get better, it's healthier for her.

The doctors are hopeful, so it's not unrealistic to believe that her father, who has a very treatable cancer, which they found early, can go into full remission. Helping Jessie grow her hope muscle, I shared hopeful stories, helped her connect with other children whose parents are in remission, and helped her do the Wheel of Feel, pivoting from where she is toward more positive feelings, including hope.

Insecurity (-)

The feeling of doubt. The emotionally healthy child is learning how to handle challenging emotions such as doubt and uncertainty without spinning into overwhelm and panic. By the nature of being on this planet, feeling doubtful about our ability to do certain things is natural, but it is not necessarily helpful. *Insecurity* is another word that means lack of confidence, certainty, or assuredness.

Learning how to overcome a lack of confidence helps a child move toward emotional balance.

Tools

- *Self-Talk:* Create mottos, and learn from others how to verbally "pump yourself up."

- *Self-Perception:* See yourself succeeding, and get the real-life opportunity to do so (see "Confidence").
- *Wisdom teachings:* Confidence list (below)

Similar Emotions

Lack of confidence, doubt, uncertainty, shakiness, nervousness

Scenario

George, age nine, is unsure of his ability to be a Wise Man in his school's Nativity play. He has to memorize his lines, wear the school costume, and not mess up. His mom, Beth, called me to see if I could help bolster his confidence and help him feel more secure because she wants to see her son feel good about himself.

Working with George, we made a "confidence list" of all the things he had successfully achieved, which he couldn't list at first, from scoring the winning soccer goal to creating his own robot at STEM (science, technology, engineering, and math) camp. In our work together, I helped George realize that feeling unsure is normal and healthy, especially when we haven't done something before, but I also helped him find the courage to try to believe that he can do it.

George also came up with some mottos: "I am the wise one, king of rocks, and I can do this!"

Love (+)

The feeling of intense like. The emotionally healthy child is learning how to love herself and others in a healthy way. Love is constructive and is present in healthy friendships, in family relationships, in community relationships such as with teachers, and even in children's relationships with their pets. Helping children learn how to think loving thoughts and feel affection is central to helping them become emotionally healthier and, ultimately, happier.

Ensuring that your child knows he or she is loved unconditionally is also part of raising an emotionally healthy child. Some boys and girls mistakenly believe they're loved only if they receive good grades or accomplish some sort of task.

Tools

- *Self-Talk:* For example, your child can say, "I love you" when she looks in the mirror at herself. Then she can say, "I really love you" and can look in her own eyes.
- *Connection:* Help your child make friendships that help her feel loved.
- *Wisdom teachings:* For example, Mother Teresa said, "Let us always meet each other with a smile, for a smile is the beginning of love."

Similar Emotions

Fondness, affection, care, unconditional positive regard

Scenario

One of my clients, Scout, says, "I hate myself" frequently. His mom, Mary Ellen, was concerned upon hearing this, which prompted her to call me. Love isn't simply about loving others but learning to love yourself and not put too much pressure on yourself. Scout got straight As in school, but when he did something wrong he would say mean things to himself, which wasn't emotionally healthy.

Learning to love yourself, as the Justin Bieber song suggests, isn't simply about having loving parents but giving that love to yourself. At my suggestion, Scout began journaling, took tae kwon do, and found mentors to help him love himself more. He even started picking friends whom he noticed were kind to themselves so he can learn how to do that better himself.

Peace (+)

The feeling of serenity. The emotionally healthy child is learning not only how to self-soothe and calm before responding to big emotions but also how to become quiet and peaceful. Children who know peace can extend peace to others. They're learning how to have a more positive emotional set point versus simply being reactive and combative.

If a whole generation of children were taught peacemaking skills, the world would likely be a more harmonious place.

Tools

- *Centering:* Mindful Meditation on page 132, Insight Timer or Headspace (free apps), or Mindful Seeing on page 119
- *Yoga:* Child's Pose (see page 159), and for others read *Yoga for Children* by Lisa Flynn
- *Wisdom Teachings:* For example, Eckhart Tolle said, "You find peace not by rearranging the circumstances of your life, but by realizing who you are at the deepest level."

Similar Emotions

Calm, feeling untroubled, feeling undisturbed, serenity, quiet, stillness

Scenario

Children are often on the move, and helping them slow down to feel peaceful can be powerful. They can connect with that place within of stillness, quiet, and serenity, which they'll need throughout their lives, since this world isn't always peaceful or easy.

Tashi, a five-year-old, is the biggest troublemaker on the playground. He was raised Buddhist, but regardless of his family's spiritual practices, he likes to pick fights. The good news is that he goes to a local Montessori school, which just began teaching a peace curriculum focused on calm and cooperation.

At first Tashi didn't want to participate, but he did enjoy child's pose and archer pose, which helped him feel calm. Soon he was doing the Tummy Time breathing meditation, which helped him feel calmer and peaceful. With breathing and movement practices, Tashi stopped picking fights and began to choose peace more often.

Sadness (-)

The feeling of being unhappy. The emotionally healthy child needs to find an outlet to release his or her sadness constructively to return to balance. Of course, sadness is a healthy emotion, especially after a loss, disappointment, or change. If your child cannot get unstuck from sadness, consider getting him or her professional assistance.

Tools

- *Awareness:* Tool 8 (Iceberg), on page 94
- *Connection:* Tool 10 (Connect Four) and Tool 7 (Smart Choices Checklist). Saying the simple words "I am here for you" can help immensely.

- *Outlets:* Tool 11 (Color It Out) or another activity (either physical or creative)
- *Pivot toward positive:* Tool 6 (Wheel of Feel), and Tool 9 (Rearview Mirror)

Similar Emotions

Misery, despair, hopelessness, loneliness, feeling rejected

Scenario

Anandhi, a mom from India, has a very holistic approach to helping her daughter, Diya, process her sadness. She does a body scan with Diya to see where she is feeling sadness and asks her to name her sadness (Tool 8). Diya says, "I feel sad in my tummy," and then they rub her tummy. They attune and connect together on what's happening. Diya continues to share that she's sad because her best friend, Megan, is moving to England that week.

Being able to be with your child, acknowledge how she feels, and help her move forward to release her feelings constructively is the goal. After Diya felt a little bit better, Anandhi set up her daughter's favorite watercolors and encouraged her to paint out her feelings. Diya painted a butterfly, which she's going to give to Megan so Megan will never forget her. It is vital that we teach children to constructively let out emotions, especially sadness, so they can regain their balance and learn that it's natural to feel sad sometimes.

Scared (−)

The feeling of fear. The emotionally healthy child feels fear and uses it as a force for good. He may decide that his fear of a certain block is smart and doesn't walk down it alone or that he can overcome his fear of, say, performing onstage. Helping your child learn to spot fear and navigate this uncomfortable emotion is essential to bringing him back to emotional balance.

Feeling fear is part of the human experience, and learning to spot it and what it means is essential.

Tools

- *Breathing:* Mindful Breathing (Five for Five) on page 117, Tool 4 (Bubble Breathing), and Tool 5 (Hand on Heart)
- *Self-Talk:* Create a motto such as "I am safe," and say it repeatedly.
- *Connection:* Being with someone who isn't afraid can reduce your child's fear, and saying, "I'm here for you" can immediately help.

Similar Emotions

Fright, fear, worry, uneasiness, dread

Scenario

Suki, age eight, is afraid at night, especially of sleeping in her own bed. Her mom and dad have tried what they say is "everything" to help her. Meeting with Suki, I discovered that she was afraid of the sounds in her room, that she only had one little light, and that she kept thinking of this scary trailer she saw for the Disney movie, *Coco*, which takes place in the land of the dead.

Since *our thoughts create our feelings,* Suki was getting stuck in her fear and what-if scenarios, wondering, *What's that sound outside? What's the shadow by the door?* Her mind was spinning, and she kept getting herself worked up. First, we worked on breathing to calm (Tool 4, Bubble Breathing) and then saying, "I am safe" as much as she needed to, along with getting her room to feel safe for her.

Helping Suki calm and begin choosing more helpful thoughts ("I am safe") and giving her some mindful tools was the first step toward bringing her back to her safe, present moment, where she could start to lessen her fears.

Selfishness (-)

The feeling of self-centeredness. The emotionally healthy child is learning how to identify and express emotions constructively while also tuning in to the emotions of others. Too much focus solely on your own needs without consideration for others is selfish, which causes other mental and emotional problems — and, ultimately, suffering.

Young children begin their lives focused on themselves, which is normal and healthy, but as maturation and emotional growth occur, the emotionally healthy child learns to expand his or her worldview to include others.

Tools

- *Mindfulness:* Practice giving to others using exercises such as Mindful Goodness on page 130.
- *Helping others*
- *Mentoring and wisdom teachings:* For example, it's scientifically proven that giving and sharing boosts happiness, which children often don't realize.

Similar Emotions

Greed, self-centeredness, and self-absorption

Scenario

Jenny doesn't want to share her toys, which is perfectly normal for a two-year-old, but her older sister, Cybil, is seven and doesn't want to share, either. Their mom, Bessy, said, "I understand Jenny is young, but Cybil doesn't have any friends. No one wants to play with her because she only cares about herself."

Children like Cybil don't yet realize that being solely focused on themselves is going to cause them pain and prevent good things from happening. Cybil and I talked about how being selfish often makes people unhappy, while thinking about or helping others makes people happier. Helping her connect the dots and start extending her circle of interest beyond herself required a three-prong approach: mentoring, helping others, and mindful exercises.

Stress (-)

The feeling of pressure. The emotionally healthy child is learning how to handle stress in healthy ways such as forming healthy habits like exercise, connection with others, good time management, and creative endeavors. Unhealthy habits would include addictive video gaming, incessant texting, and binge-watching television for days.

Some things that stress children out include: preschoolers being left at school (separation anxiety), middle-school applications, school dances, sports tryouts, changing schools, taking timed exams, television shows (when they're scary or inappropriate), seeing the news, and extreme weather (hurricanes, wildfires).

Tools

- *Calming:* Tool 4 (Bubble Breathing), Tool 5 (Hand on Heart), and Mindful Breathing (Five for Five), on page 117

- *Outlets:* Exercise that makes you sweat is particularly de-stressing.
- *Creative endeavors:* Finding something that relaxes your children, whether it's reading or playing in a sandbox, is essential.

Similar Emotions

Pressure, anxiety, worry, uncertainty, fear

Scenario

Josie, age fourteen, was stressed about college applications and was putting a great deal of pressure on herself. She says, "I want to be a pediatrician" while continuing to tell me she needs straight As, and she gets very little sleep because of her self-imposed stress. Of course, the problem with stress is it doesn't actually help you get better grades or perform better. Some pressure or deadlines may help us accomplish things, but carrying the weight of the world does not.

Connecting with Josie, I helped her take some pressure off herself by having her focus on the present moment with awareness. We did several rounds of Mindful Breathing, we loaded the Insight Timer app onto her phone, and we meditated together. The goal was to help Josie find her center of calmness and connect there.

Worry (-)

The feeling of concern. The emotionally healthy child is learning to be mindful, which means present and aware of what's happening now. Children who worry tend to be highly intelligent but nervous or anxious. They see the possibilities of something bad happening in the future or feel nervous about the past, but they're not in the present moment.

Worrying is greatly influenced by our genes. That's not to say that if you worry, your children will worry, but the propensity will be there. This is helpful because knowing that there's biology involved in worry, anxiety, and nervousness makes it less personal.

Tools

- *Mindfulness:* Mindful Breathing, on page 116, and deliberate self talk, such as, "I am safe" and "all is well" can help.
- *Worry-reduction exercises:* Tool 6 (Wheel of Feel), exercises (below)
- *Wisdom teachings:* For example, the Dalai Lama always says, "If a problem is fixable, if a situation is such that you can do something about it, then there is no need to worry. If it's not fixable, then there is no help in worrying. There is no benefit in worrying whatsoever."

Similar Emotions

Nervousness, anxiety, fear, stress, concern

Scenario

Lauren, mom of tween Harry, struggles with how to help him manage his worry and enjoy his life more. On the airplane with his family, Harry asked, "Have you ever crash-landed? Do terrorists still get on planes? What happens if we die?" He spins the what-if scenarios until he's almost in a full panic, which negatively impacts everyone's mood on the way to their annual vacation to Disney World in Florida.

To help her son, Lauren focuses on what we now know — the pilots have training, there is trained security, and every day planes fly safely. This eases her son a bit, and she also began using my Wheel of Feel (Tool 6) as a refocusing tool to pivot Harry toward the positive. Instead of feelings, she used sayings, such as "I am now safe," "JFK is safe," "I love Florida," and "My favorite ride is Space Mountain," and slowly he started moving in a new direction.

Helping children reduce worry is always about bringing them back to the present moment and creating secure and safe ways to handle the unknown. Some parents even say, "You have ten minutes to worry, and when the time is up, the worrying must end." Surprisingly, this often works to contain anxiety.

Along with "Worry Time" from her book *Why Smart Kids Worry*, Allison Edwards offers another idea, which is to limit your child to five questions so they cannot endlessly spin on their worry, creating a worry storm. I love this idea because it helps children release their thoughts and helps them come back to the present, mindful, and perhaps less worrisome moment.

TAKE NOTE

MEDIA AND WORRY

Like adults, children are susceptible to seeing media images and feeling worry as well as stress. They get addicted to what's happening, which creates a bump of feel-good chemicals in their brain but also physical stress, especially if there is troubling news, whether it's a mudslide in California or a missing person in New Jersey.

When children are exposed to too much media, especially news programs, many begin to feel stressed and expect things to go wrong. In other words, they're looking for things to worry about, which doesn't help them.

Raising a media-healthy child today is more complex than ever, but mentoring, moderation, and age-appropriate access to information are essential to helping him or her feel safe in this sometimes unsettling world, especially online.

Beyond the Basics

It is our responsibility to learn to become emotionally intelligent. These are skills, they're not easy, nature didn't give them to us — we have to learn them.

PAUL EKMAN

With this toolbox, my goal is to give you a starting point to help your children with their big emotions, such as anger, sadness, stress, and worry, while also proactively cultivating habits for emotional health, such as gratitude and generosity. With this toolbox we can help our children:

- identify their emotions
- develop an emotional language to communicate these emotions
- use tools to constructively express their emotions
- steer themselves toward positive emotional health

Beyond the emotions in the toolbox, there are many more emotions felt by our children regularly, such as surprise, delight, disgust, boredom, fatigue, jealousy, silliness, revenge, and embarrassment. One of my middle-school clients, Maya, tells me that she's embarrassed every day by her parents and feels bored daily at school. Children like Maya have opportunities every day to increase their discomfort tolerance, whether it's when Mom is saying something uncool or they're sitting through a dry subject like American history.

American psychologist Paul Ekman also found six core emotions across the world: anger, disgust, fear, happiness, sadness, and surprise. Two of the emotions I didn't include in the toolbox are disgust and surprise. Of course, it's easy to see how our children regularly experience surprise, from opening a gift under the Christmas tree to playing hide and seek. But disgust is more complicated, from my perspective. Disgust is the feeling of extreme disapproval, which children experience especially when they're asked to eat something they hate. It creates immediate imbalances and suffering in children.

As you can see, children feel many emotions — some of them bringing them closer to health and wellness, some steering them away from their joy.

Coming Back to Balance

When we have a good balance between thinking and feeling
...our actions and lives are always the richer for it.

YO-YO MA

Coming back to emotional balance is something we practice throughout our lives, but children who begin earlier have more time getting it right and potentially with more ease. Of course, anger, sadness, loss, and disappointment are never easy at any point in life's journey, but learning how to navigate these emotions early on is helpful. Said differently, many of today's children have the chance to grow up emotionally healthy, and that can only be a good thing.

Becoming emotionally healthier isn't just about managing challenging emotions but, as we've been discussing, it includes:

- cultivating a positive mindset
- being mindful
- developing character
- creating healthy habits

A positive and optimistic person learns how to perpetually turn lemons into lemonade, but you don't need to be all sunny sunshine to be emotionally healthy. That's part temperament. Being able to grow up emotionally healthier means you're learning not only to identify your emotions but also to pause before reacting to them — especially the fast-moving and challenging ones — and, ultimately, to make smarter choices.

Emotional health and wholeness are about the choices we make and the ones we help our children make. Children are always faced with choices, such as whether to tease the new kid in class or cheat on their spelling exam — or to hold the door open for their friend or smile at the crossing guard. Even little choices, when they're smart ones, can help them lift their mood and brighten their day.

Emotional Coaching: The Top Five

If children feel safe, they can take risks; ask questions, make mistakes, learn to trust, share their feelings, and grow.

ALFIE KOHN

Coaching your child on his or her emotions can be tricky, but it's the work of modern parents, especially those wanting to raise emotionally healthy children. Of course, some children are easier than others regarding emotional outbursts, proclivity toward anger or sadness, or problematic behaviors, but with time, tools, and practice progress can be made. I can also say that the best emotional coaches do certain things, which I list as my *Top Five* pointers:

1. Connect.
2. Be a calming presence.
3. Listen fully.
4. Focus on problem solving (not punishment).
5. Learn together.

In addition, over and over I hear from children how words hurt or help them heal in emotional moments. I see children hang on my words. Although I couldn't even remember what game I played with Jenny last Tuesday, for her it was life changing. After she got home she had her mother order the game, *Clue*, and has been practicing all week to beat me and show me how good she's gotten.

Children are impressionable, which sounds obvious, but they're literally creating how they feel about themselves and their world through what we say and the messages we send them. They want to feel seen, heard, and safe while being able to explore and discover their interests with gusto. I remember being a young child and having a "flashbulb moment" when someone said something that changed my self-perception, and I remember everything about that moment — for better or worse. Of course, our aim is to give our children positive flashbulb moments, to the best of our ability.

Almost Done

We've traveled together through these chapters, deepening our understanding of what emotional health and wholeness look like.

There have likely been moments of frustration when I've asked you to step up and do something different, as well as moments of recognition when you see you've been doing everything right in helping your son or daughter. It's not an all-or-nothing proposition but a process of becoming our emotional best and helping our children do the same.

Chapter Seven

PROGRESS, NOT PERFECTION

Everybody's a work in progress. I'm a work in progress. I've never arrived....I'm still learning all the time.

RENÉE FLEMING

In my first real job, I remember sitting in my corporate office and sending an email when I was feeling angry. Before long my boss, Rich, who was the CEO, called me into his office and said, "Maureen, I need you to employ the twenty-four-hour rule." Not knowing what this rule was, I inquired, and Rich explained his request for me to wait twenty-four hours before responding to any email that got me annoyed or angry. I quickly agreed, since I was only twenty-two years old and wanted to keep my first professional job. Little did I know that after twenty-four hours, my anger always dissipated and I could respond calmly. This was progress.

Children make progress incrementally, too, especially as they become emotionally healthier. One day your child stops pushing his sibling and instead walks away stomping his feet when he's angry. Not perfect, but certainly progress. Our goal in raising emotionally healthy children is to guide them to recognize emotions, help them understand what they can do to cope with them, and help them make better choices. It doesn't mean your child goes from major tantrums to tantrum-free in thirty days — although that's possible. What it does mean is that with help, things get better.

My client Max, age eight, is a perfect example. He came to me earlier in the year because of his anger issues at school. Angela, his mom, was exhausted from getting urgent calls from the principal. As a single mother whose stress was understandably at an all-time high, she needed assistance. Connecting with Max, I realized he had unresolved grief about his dad dying two years earlier, and his anger issues only emerged during the month his school was celebrating dads (ouch). So I helped Max constructively express his deep feelings and learn new tools for handling his anger, which moved him in a positive direction.

What I know for sure is that today's children are smarter than ever and can learn how to handle their emotions. Because they're small and new to the world, children simply don't know what they don't know, but with intelligent instruction, tools, and practice, the sky's the limit. And a little guidance can go a long way, so start where you are, and before you know it, progress will happen.

The Emotionally Healthy Child

Your emotions follow your thoughts just as surely as baby ducks follow their mother.

DAVID D. BURNS

Children developing emotional balance are learning how to regulate their bodies and emotions, which begins with their thoughts.

They are starting to see that they're bigger than their biggest emotions and that they're in charge. Bae, one of my child clients, loves to say, "I'm the boss, applesauce," to remind himself he's in charge, even when he feels angry, frustrated, or annoyed with someone.

Guiding children on the path of positive emotional health, and helping them learn the skill of balance, means we're helping them acquire:

- cognitive control
- emotional awareness (knowledge)
- self-control (behavior modification)
- decision-making abilities

Ultimately, we want to help our children make smart choices, even when they're experiencing challenging emotions like frustration, disgust, or anger. The more practice boys and girls have at expressing emotions constructively — especially the trickiest ones like anger, which are so fast-moving — the better they can do in the moment when you're not around and they want to push someone on the playground. Through practice, they learn how to walk away and make a smarter choice.

Something I tell children is that it's okay to want to hit someone, but hitting someone is not acceptable (unless, of course, it's in self-defense). There really are no unhealthy emotions, but it's what we do with them that matters. As I mentioned in chapter 2, more helpful emotions like compassion and gratitude naturally move your children toward emotional balance, while challenging emotions like jealousy and anger move them away from balance. So along with handling challenging emotions, we want to help our children cultivate positive inner qualities and emotions like compassion, kindness, and generosity, which mightily move them toward well-being.

The Emotional Health Equation

Just as your car runs more smoothly and requires less energy to go faster and farther when the wheels are in perfect alignment, you perform better when your thoughts, feelings, emotions, goals, and values are in balance.

BRIAN TRACY

Children are all different, especially in their personalities and emotional proclivities. It's no surprise that some tend toward sadness and others have happy-go-lucky personalities. But no matter what your children's unique personality and emotional needs are, they need you to connect and emotionally coach them toward self-mastery.

Throughout this book, we've discussed the different pieces of the emotional health puzzle, which are:

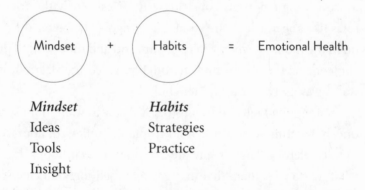

Mindset	*Habits*
Ideas	Strategies
Tools	Practice
Insight	

Children are learning how emotions work (chapter 3), what to do with the challenging ones and how to create helpful ones (chapter 4), and the power of paying attention to their bodies and feelings (chapter 5) in becoming emotionally healthy. They're having the *direct experiences* of putting new ideas and tools into practice as well as refining how they move themselves toward better feelings.

Beyond the mindset of emotional health are the habits or practices that when done regularly can pave positive pathways in your children's developing brains. Instead of defaulting to a knee-jerk reaction such as screaming, they learn, for example, that they can take a mindful moment or shoot hoops in the backyard.

This simple equation of mindset plus habits equals emotional health is the starting point for helping your children move from reactivity to responsiveness, rigidity to flexibility, and carelessness to careful choices. It sets a path where you now know where you're going and can help get your children moving with you in that direction, hopefully with more ease.

Habits Create Health

We are what we repeatedly do.

WILL DURANT

Creating habits can help us move toward any goal, whether it's building muscles at the gym or learning how to calm and center. The power of habit is immeasurable. In her book *Better Than Before*, Gretchen Rubin shares how habits change our lives little by little, especially when we schedule those habits. What I know for sure is that creating habits such as my Five Joys before bedtime every night lifts my heart and helps my mind focus on the good things. It's a simple practice but something I do without even thinking because it's become a habit.

When we do something regularly without needing to think about it, it becomes a habit. Let me give you another example. I love coffee, but the doctor said it's not good for my body (ugh). To help myself quit the coffee habit and replace it with a healthier one, I place two lemons nightly in the kitchen, and when I wake I make a hot lemon concoction with cayenne. So I replaced my coffee habit with something better for my body, and boom — it happens daily without much thought. I have simply taken my thoughts, my mind, out of the equation and harnessed the power of habit.

Although I have encouraged the development of mind*ful*ness in children and ourselves, there is also a powerful ally in mind-*less*ness. Habits help us take our resistance and our minds out of the equation. The ability to create a habit helps us not overthink something, and whether it's hitting the gym or doing a gratitude or breathing exercise with our children, it gets hardwired into our lives.

Creating habits of positive emotional health with our children can help them master their emotions and become happier. Some of these include:

- *Bedtime ritual.* Hand on Heart (Tool 5) is used by many of my clients to help their children associate relaxation and calm with this gesture, which helps them calm in their emotional moments.
- *After-school activity.* In chapter 5, Hana helped her children feel gratitude daily by sitting cross-legged on the ground and going around the room tapping their hearts, then saying what they were grateful for from that day.
- *Mindfulness.* Elementary school teacher Liz Slade guides her students to do a calming exercise after recess to settle down and reconnect with the present moment.

Children build their lives on what we show them, the words we say to them, and the habits we help them create. It's up to us to help them build healthier habits, especially around how to stop, calm, and bring themselves back to emotional balance. Regular habits, not periodic ones, are important to nurture in children. They help children acquire the ability to calm faster despite whatever may be happening, and then come back to their center.

My suggestion is to choose one thing and incorporate it into your emotional health program. Whether that is meditating together or practicing daily gratitude, there really is great power in adding one thing. Before you know it, things change and progress happens. One family I know added a Peace Corner in their house, so when their children were upset they could go to that corner, which was full of books, stuffed animals, art, and games, to calm themselves and regain their center. One time, five-year-old Samuel told his mom when she was angry, "Mom, I think you need five minutes in the Peace Corner," and she chuckled because it was true.

TAKE NOTE

THE FOUR SKILLS

Cultivating the four emotional skills we discussed in chapter 2 helps children to catch themselves, stop, calm, and then make smarter choices. Specifically, children are learning to:

- pay attention
- press pause
- respond (vs. react)
- make a smart choice

Each of these skills is something to develop in your children, a process that can be helped along by mindfulness practices and role-modeling. I do believe in the saying "Give your child something good to imitate," because imitate they will do. The good news is that your healthy children have the capability to pay attention, stop, and then respond instead of simply reacting negatively to situations. I suggest picking one of these four skills and focusing on it for a month with your children. You may be amazed by how soon they shift their behavior.

Three Steps to Success

*Success is nothing more than a few simple disciplines, prac-
ticed every day.*

JIM ROHN

In review, the main thing I want you to take away from our journey are the three steps to success. Each step could fill a book, but
I have simplified them so we can teach and role-model them to
our children:

1. stop
2. calm
3. make a smart choice

Stop: Children, as you know, move quickly, and helping them
slow down and stop is the first step in helping them change emotional directions. The emotion may be something helpful like excitement, but too much of it can cause them to knock something
over in the dining room, so the three steps are for emotions that
are both helpful and challenging. Of course, when children experience challenging emotions, it's essential to slow their momentum and help them steer their emotional boat in a new, healthier
direction.

Calm: Calming is something we learn throughout our lives, but
certainly the things that helped me calm as a child still help me
calm as an adult. Remember, you are helping your children build
lifelong tools of calming and centering. I grew up on the East
Coast, and I would go into nature to feel calm, and today, on the
West Coast, that still remains my number one way to feel relaxed
(besides meditation and laughter). While I may have climbed

more trees when I was little, today when I have all ten toes in the sand, my stress lifts off instantly.

Make a smart choice: Along with stopping and calming, the ability to make a smart choice is essential. Whether a child decides to scream or take deep breaths, push her sister or use her words, or throw a book across the room or walk away, these choices all have an impact. Choices are best made when the emotional intensity of a situation has lessened, which is why step 2, calm, precedes making a smart choice.

Choices that are good for you and good for others are smart choices. Although I am specifically talking about emotionally charged choices, they can really be choices about anything in life. If your child was planning her birthday party list, she could think about what she'd like to eat and what others would enjoy, too — and that's a smart choice.

Emotional Growth

Do the best you can until you know better. Then when you know better, do better.

MAYA ANGELOU

Coaching our children to recognize their emotions, learn to calm, and then make better choices when feeling a big emotion is growth. It may be messy and ugly in moments, but it's what growth looks like. Just like the lotus seed, which goes through the dirt and pushes up through water to flower, we have to go through the dirt of our lives in order to bloom. The same is true for children and for us, as we help them grow into the people they were born to be.

Sometimes we think growth is supposed to be simple and easy, but most often it looks like this:

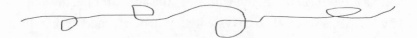

Charlie may be crying every time you drop him off at school and needing you to walk him to the door, even though he's nine years old. Then there comes a moment when Charlie says, "Mom, I'm good," and he doesn't need you anymore — especially after learning deep breaths, creating some mottos, and doing some confidence-building exercises (see my book *Growing Happy Kids*). Growth often feels like three steps forward, two steps back, three steps forward; it is by no means a forward march but more like the cha-cha.

One way to nurture emotional growth in children is to help them see that whatever they send out gets returned to them in some way, shape, or form. For example, if they treat someone unkindly, something unkind will likely be returned to them. Children who learn about this boomerang effect naturally want to send good things into the universe, which means they'll get good (emotionally speaking) things back in return. As adults we know it as the law of cause and effect, but using the term *boomerang* is a great way to explain it. (Buddhists call it your enlightened self-interest, which recognizes that by being good, you allow better things to flow into your life.)

So in the process of raising emotionally healthy children, we need to stay flexible and steadfast in our commitment to helping them learn skills of emotional health, even when it's messy and challenging. Because it's never a straight line, but forward, backward, sideways and then sometimes a quantum leap. Our goal is to be there for our children in guiding them and growing together.

Learning Together

I am still learning.

MICHELANGELO, AT AGE EIGHTY-SEVEN

Coaching children on their emotions requires that we get (or keep) our emotional house in order as well as cut ourselves some slack. No one is perfect, and we're all learning. Some days we're learning patience, tolerance, and forgiveness, while other days we're learning about laughter and joy. The lessons are constant, but the rewards are great when raising today's children to be who they came here to be.

What I see from my vantage point is that the best parents, teachers, and adults learn alongside children and don't have any trouble saying, "I don't know" if they sincerely don't know, but instead they seek to learn together. For example, Autumn, at age eight recently lost one of her best friends to cancer, and her mom said, "Honey, I don't know why this happened." Her mom didn't give her a fake explanation but decided to be honest and offer her sincere comfort while helping her work through her grief.

The process of learning together also means that we may make mistakes with our children, but we can repair the parent-child relationship when that happens. One dad I know sometimes lets curses fly in the car, and his son thinks it's hysterical, but the father makes sure to tell his son those words are not to be repeated, and he apologizes to him. Learning together has many facets, including:

- repairing the parent-child relationship (when emotional mishaps occur)
- focusing on partnership (versus punishment)
- being honest (in age-appropriate ways)
- being authentic
- having fun

All these facets are part of learning about how emotions work, what you can do to feel better today, and how to develop the inner qualities that draw happier experiences into your life. Because in general the better you feel, the better things go.

Till Next Time

Happy trails to you, until we meet again.

DALE EVANS

Today's children are powerful creators, and they have the capacity to create well-being for themselves, sooner rather than later. They simply need the ideas, tools, and practice, along with wise instruction and mentors, to coach them into their greatness. They can be good on their own, but to be truly great, compassionate, and kind beings in a sometimes not-so-kind world takes courage, inner confidence (or as many say, grit), and a community of healthy people saying, "Come this way."

On our journey together, I hope you've been awakened to your greatness, too. The role of parents, educators, and other caring adults is enormous. This includes raising and role-modeling positive emotional health, even through the tough times. But when we know the truth — that we are deliberate creators and that our emotions follow our thoughts — we become mindful about what we focus on.

My wish for you is that you get the opportunity to focus on joyful experiences with your children as they grow into healthier, happier, and whole beings. They're on their way, but whether today is an easy or challenging day, growth happens step-by-step. What I do promise you is that every experience, even the ones that feel like mud, can be fertile soil in which to plant your child's healthier and happier life.

GRATITUDE

Thank you to my teachers. Those who came in big bodies and those who came in small ones. I feel genuinely blessed to learn and, in turn, to teach others.

Specific appreciation goes to my literary agent, Lilly Ghahremani, who helped me envision a bigger and grander life for this book. My long-term editor, Candace Johnson, who I hope no one discovers, is incredible and talented beyond words. Of course, the team at New World Library, specifically Jason Gardner, my acquiring editor, has been a joy to work with. I also deeply appreciate the many people who encouraged me throughout the writing of this book, from Jim at La Casa de Maria to my sister, Trish, mom of three beautiful girls.

My gratitude wouldn't be complete if I didn't thank the parents and children I work with. They let me into their lives and trusted me to help them on their journey. For that I'm incredibly grateful, and I feel blessed to be on this path with you.

Generosity

One of my teachers used to say, "If you have the opportunity to be generous, take it," and that made an impression on me. The giving doesn't have to be money; it can be a kind word, a smile, or a helping hand when someone needs it.

In the spirit of generosity, I'm giving 10 percent of my author proceeds to help children's health initiatives around the world so that more children have the opportunity for health and happiness. Specific organizations I am supporting include Vitamin Angels and Direct Relief.

RESOURCES

Books

Ben-Shahar, Tal. *Choose the Life You Want: The Mindful Way to Happiness*. New York: The Experiment, 2012.

Borba, Michele. *UnSelfie: Why Empathetic Kids Succeed in Our All-About-Me World*. New York: Touchstone/Simon & Schuster, 2016.

Burns, David D. *Feeling Good: The New Mood Therapy*. New York: HarperCollins, 2008.

Carter, Christine. *Raising Happiness: 10 Simple Steps for More Joyful Kids and Happier Parents*. New York: Ballantine Books, 2010.

Dalai Lama, Tutu, Desmond, and Douglas Abrams. *The Book of Joy: Lasting Happiness in a Changing World*. New York: Avery, 2016.

Duckworth, Angela. *Grit: The Power of Passion and Perseverance*. New York: Scribner, 2016.

Dunckley, Victoria. *Reset Your Child's Brain: A Four-Week Plan to End Meltdowns, Raise Grades, and Boost Social Skills by Reversing the*

Effects of Electronic Screen-Time. Novato, CA: New World Library, 2015.

Dweck, Carol. *Mindset: The New Psychology of Success*. New York: Ballantine, 2006.

Edwards, Allison. *Why Smart Kids Worry: And What Parents Can Do to Help*. Naperville, IL: Sourcebooks, 2013.

Flynn, Lisa. *Yoga for Children: 200+ Yoga Poses, Breathing Exercises, and Meditations for Healthier, Happier, More Resilient Children*. Avon, MA: Adams Media, 2013.

Hanh, Thich Nhat. *You Are Here: Discovering the Magic of the Present Moment*. Berkeley, CA: Parallax, 2010.

———. *No Mud, No Lotus: The Art of Transforming Suffering*. Berkeley, CA: Parallax, 2014.

———. *The Art of Living: Peace and Freedom in the Here and Now*. New York: HarperCollins, 2017.

Healy, Maureen. *Growing Happy Kids: How to Foster Inner Confidence, Success, and Happiness*. Deerfield Beach, FL: HCI Books, 2012.

———. *The Energetic Keys to Indigo Kids: Your Guide to Raising and Resonating with the New Children*. Pompton Plains, NJ: New Page Books, 2013.

Heitner, Devorah. *Screenwise: Helping Kids Thrive (and Survive) in Their Digital World*. Brookline, MA: Bibliomotion, 2016.

Kabat-Zinn, Jon. *Wherever You Go, There You Are: Mindfulness Meditation in Everyday Life*. New York: Hachette, 2005.

———. *Full Catastrophe Living: Using the Wisdom of Your Body and Mind to Face Stress, Pain, and Illness*. New York: Bantam, 2013.

Kohn, Alfie. *The Schools Our Children Deserve: Moving Beyond Traditional Classrooms and "Tougher Standards."* New York: Mariner Books, 2000.

———. *Feel-Bad Education: And Other Contrarian Essays on Children and Schooling*. Boston, MA: Beacon Press, 2011.

Ricard, Matthieu. *Happiness: A Guide to Developing Life's Most Important Skill*. New York: Little Brown, 2006.

Salzberg, Sharon. *Real Happiness: The Power of Meditation*. New York: Workman, 2011.

Siegel, Daniel J., and Tina Payne Bryson. *The Whole-Brain Child: 12 Revolutionary Strategies to Nurture Your Child's Developing Mind.* New York: Bantam, 2012.

———. *The Yes Brain: How to Cultivate Courage, Curiosity, and Resilience in Your Child.* New York: Bantam, 2018.

Stabile, Scott. *Big Love: The Power of Living with a Wide-Open Heart.* Novato, CA: New World Library, 2017.

Tolle, Eckhart. *The Power of Now: A Guide to Spiritual Enlightenment.* Novato, CA: New World Library, 1999.

Online Sources

Gelles, David. "Mindfulness for Children." *New York Times.* Accessed November 15, 2017. https://www.nytimes.com/guides/well /mindfulness-for-children.

Gerszberg, Caren Osten. "The Future of Education, Mindful Classrooms." *Mindful.* Accessed December 2, 2017. https://www.mindful .org/mindfulness-in-education.

Healy, Maureen. "Forgiveness: Are You Really Teaching Your Kids How to Forgive?" *Psychology Today.* September 27, 2010. https://www .psychologytoday.com/us/blog/creative-development/201009 /forgiveness.

INDEX

ABOUT THE AUTHOR

Maureen Healy is a sought-after speaker, educator, and leader in the field of children's emotional health. Her first book, *Growing Happy Kids*, won the 2014 Nautilus and Readers' Favorite book awards. Maureen also writes a popular blog for *Psychology Today* and has contributed to the PBS series "This Emotional Life."

Unique about Maureen is her experience working with children worldwide, from northern India to northern California. Her expertise in social and emotional learning has taken her throughout the United States, Europe, and Asia. Currently, Maureen is based in Santa Barbara, California, where she continues to work with educators, parents, and their children.

Maureen received a BA in psychology and an MBA from Clark University in Worcester, Massachusetts; she also completed her PhD coursework in child psychology from Fielding Graduate University in Santa Barbara, California. Along with these traditional credentials, Maureen has traveled the world studying happiness with well-known teachers, which has bolstered her joy immensely. To learn more, go to www.growinghappykids.com.